A Crazy Quilt Life

A Crazy Quilt Life

A Memoir

Sherry Comstock

Sherry Comstock

To my cherished husband, Keith, my champion through all my incarnations.

To my children, James, David, Kenny and Sarah, each of you helps to focus the lens through which I view the world.

To Carolyn T. Davis, Momma, for everything.

Other than my family, I have changed created composites for or changed the names of individuals in this book. The thoughts, memories are mine. I have endeavored not to tell anyone else's story.

CONTENTS

CONTENTS

CONTENTS

Prologue

"Hey, Momma! How's it going?" Kenny asked, bending his tall frame to give me a hug. *How tall he's gotten. My head doesn't even reach his shoulders.*

"It's so good to see you! Come see what I've done in the library." We left the kitchen and went on to the library. I showed him two crazy quilt pieces I had framed.

"Did you do those?"

"No, Grandmother made them when she lived in Manassas. They're made from scraps of old suits she collected while volunteering at Serve, Prince William Hospital's auxiliary thrift store. I've carried them around for years and finally decided how to show them."

"I didn't think those were your colors. Her stitches are so small."

"I know. Such deep purples, grays, browns, and lavenders. The gorgeous hand embroidery and the play with texture, rough wools, and smooth velvets. She worked them all together. Momma was so talented and could blend colors and patterns in unexpected ways. Many times, they didn't look like they could go together."

"Where did you get them framed?"

"At Michael's, you know, the craft store. They appreciated her needlework. The sales lady kept calling the other employees over to see the pieces. We spent an hour working out how to mat and frame them. Choosing the frame was easy, but I kept adding to the matting. One mat would have been sufficient. I shouldn't have gone over my budget. I've called them Sherry's Folly."

"Why? Do you think it was silly to have them framed? I think it's outstanding. Having the two mats bring out the colors better."

"No. Remember the Reverend Mothers in Dune? They built ornamental buildings at the Chapter House that had nothing to do with the challenging times in which they worked and lived. It makes me think of Momma and how she could always create something wonderful out of nothing."

"Oh yeah, I remember. I like it!"

He turned and picked a picture of Momma holding a small baby. She is a teenager. Her head tilts down, smiling at the baby she holds facing the camera. She's pulled her long brown hair back into a neat bun. She and the baby are immaculate. Her shirtwaist dress is unwrinkled before the era of synthetic fabrics. Momma's standing in someone's backyard. The house's white paint is peeling with mostly bare board showing through. Galvanized tubs, a mop bucket and a wringer washing machine stand on the back porch.

"Is that you she's holding? She looks so young."

"I was around a month old. I'm not sure where we were, somewhere around Rock Hill or maybe Johns Island. She was only sixteen when I was born. Grandpa signed for her to get married when she was fourteen and my dad was seventeen."

"Do you think she knew what she was going to start way back then? I mean, everything she did herself and how she motivated the generations that followed her?"

"Don't know if she knew it at that moment. But she constantly pushed to 'better herself' and pushed us kids to do our best. She must have had something in mind early because she never let me pick up the Charleston accent. 'Everybody will think you're a dummy if you talk like that,' she always said."

As I reflect on that conversation with my son, I can't help but wonder how did that baby get to here...

Momma

Momma and I grew up together. She was everywhere in my childhood and most of my adulthood. The one constant through everything. Momma was always there until she wasn't. At 68 years old, she died March 4, 2007. I lost my best female friend at 52. We were fortunate; our relationship grew from mother and daughter to one of adult women.

It's hard to understand Momma, or me, unless you know something about her. She raised five children on her own. She worked until the last few years of her life. Even then she was trying to figure out eBay. Usually, she had two or three jobs. Until her brother was old enough to work, Momma was a laborer in Grandpa's construction business. Working with him, she learned to frame a house and other aspects of construction. Later, she held jobs as a waitress, a nanny, and a convenience store clerk. Eventually, she owned a store.

Through her, I learned the realities faced by women in the 1950s. She told me how my grandma was pregnant virtually every year until she contracted tuberculosis. Grandma had five living children, six stillborn babies, and who knows how many miscarriages. Because of her diabetes, Grandma had trouble carrying a baby to term. Birth control pills did not become available until 1965. Not one doctor would perform a hysterectomy or tubal ligation. They didn't think about her physical and emotional trauma. Grandma was 43 years old when she died. Momma was twenty-three.

Momma taught me so many things beyond housekeeping, child rearing, and cooking. Even before I was an adult, she was always talking to me. To some extent, I was her confidante because there was no one else around. I know she spent most of her life in sheer exhaustion. She carried a great deal of anger. She held on to anger towards people she felt had wronged her, and many had, but also towards society and the way it treats women.

Of all the things she taught me, among the two most valuable was to have an insatiable curiosity about everything around me and a drive to "improve myself", as she would have said. That drive would see me through nursing school and other challenges life sent my way. Curiosity about how my job fit in with the rest of an organization served me well throughout my professional career. Curiosity about how people from diverse cultures viewed the world helped me understand patients and neighbors. Then I'm just curious about most things. I've always wanted to understand the why.

I almost forgot pride. Pride in yourself, your work, and your home, no matter how "lowly" someone else might consider your circumstances. To find better-paying jobs, my family moved so many times I can't accurately recall all of them. Much less exactly in what order they occurred. Some were middle class; these were easier to clean. Others never lost the musky moldy smell of oldness which seeped through no matter how much you scrubbed with Pine-Sol or Clorox. "Do the best you can with what you've got," she always told us. Her pride in herself led her from small apartments and waitressing to owning her own business while raising a family. Her pride in me led me to where I am today.

Our lives are so intertwined. There's no one story that crystalizes our relationship. There were many times we disagreed. The disagreements usually occurred over raising children or me not being assertive enough.

"They'll learn faster if you'd just spank them once in a while." Momma said. Jimmy and David were small. I'd become frustrated because they kept aggravating each other and had put them in timeout.

"Spanking them will just teach them that violence is the way to solve their problems." I countered. "I don't want them to think that way."

To her credit, once I made my choice clear, she stood by my decision.

Profanity was never part of her repertoire. As she grew up, people said things like "it's enough to make a preacher cuss" or "I'm madder than a wet hen". When I was misbehaving as a child, she said "you're dancing on my last nerve". If she was talking about someone pushing her buttons, she would say something like "when they said that forty eleven hells flew right through me".

While reminiscing with Kenny, he reminded me of a time he and Sarah were watching the Price Is Right with Momma. "You called Sarah into the kitchen for something. Sarah answered you, but didn't go see what you wanted.

'Sarah, your transmission broke?' Grandmother asked in between puffs of her breathing treatment.

Sarah stopped and looked at Grandmother. But neither one of us really understood what Grandmother was saying. I kind of got that Grandmother was telling Sarah to go see you. Sarah didn't get it but figured out that the right answer was 'no ma'am'. Grandmother then tells her, 'You better get it in gear then'.

Even I didn't totally understand about the transmission and gears, but Sarah figured out quickly she needed to go see what you wanted."

As she got older, Momma developed a flamboyancy, which contrasted strongly with my childhood memories and my own understated style. Momma was always pushing me to be more assertive, to be my best. She was my loudest cheerleader.

I've never been to England or anywhere in the world of horse racing. Still, Dick Francis' exploration of family relationships always intrigued me. In *To The Hilt*, the protagonist has an epiphany concerning his relationship with his mother and how he incorporated parts of her personality into his own. To paraphrase his conclusions, that I took her pride and drive to ridiculous lengths to prove I was worthy of her efforts was "not her fault but mine."

Fans, Flowers, and Snakes

It's the fall of 2003. Momma and I are packing up the house on Marstellar Drive. She's getting ready to move to Texas. I had just finished packing up one bedroom. Thinking we should eat, I head down the hall, looking for Momma. I call out for her but don't get an answer. *Ah, there she is.* Sitting on an ottoman surrounded by boxes, she's staring at a paper in her hand.

"Look at this. Your grandmother's paystub from 1953."

I look at it in disbelief. She took home $21.34 one week after working 24 hours. Her take home pay was less than a dollar an hour. Grandma worked in the Aragon Baldwin Mills, part of J. P. Stevens in Rock Hill, SC.

"This is for real?"

"Yup, disgusting, isn't it? They blocked all the windows in those mills. When Momma came home, cotton fibers covered her like a hairnet. A ten-pound bag of sugar cost eighty-nine cents and a loaf of bread cost sixteen cents back then.

Not long after we moved to John's Island, Momma was in a TB sanitorium. She didn't stay too long because they darn near killed her by not treating her diabetes right. So, we girls took care of her at home, cooked and did the housework. Judy, BJ, and Butch were still living at home. We had a trailer right there on the property."

"A green and white one?"

"That's the one."

"It's hard to imagine trying to manage diabetes and not having a glucometer."

"We put a dipstick in her urine."

I shake my head; glad I was practicing nursing in a more modern era. "Come on, Momma, let's get some lunch."

"Okay, but you put this box in your car. There's some of my old paystubs and stuff like that in here."

Dutifully, I take the box out to the car. *I'm not sure what I'll ever do with this. I don't know how Momma hung on to it through all the moves.*

After lunch, Momma laid down to rest for a while. I return to packing, but my mind isn't on it. I try to conjure a mental picture of Grandma. With some effort, I'm four years old again and back on Johns Island...

We've gone over to Grandma's so Momma can get the laundry done. For a while I watch Momma doing laundry. She stretches Grandpa's work pants on metal frames to help shape them for ironing before putting them on the clothesline. Once she has everything hung on the clothesline, we go inside. Now she will iron the sheets, pillowcases, Grandpa's work shirts and whatever else she had washed and dried earlier while I was still sleeping. Laundry was an all-day affair. And I'm bored.

I leave Momma to the hot ironing and run to the patio. Grandma's in her chaise lounge with her *Reader's Digest* in her lap. Carefully avoiding the small brown paper bag full of tissues sitting beside her on the floor, I climb up next to Grandma. Without missing a beat, she reads aloud from the *Reader's Digest* since she finished her morning Bible study. She waits for me to pick out words I know. Grandma always smells sweet, To A Wild Rose, an Avon fragrance. A ceiling fan spins in the sweltering heat, making the patio tolerable. Today is special. We share a Hershey almond bar. I break apart the chocolate, eat it, while feeding the almonds to Grandma.

Grandma's hair is dark brown and wavy, not straight like mine would be once it grew. Like me, her eyes are dark brown, but unlike me, she is pale. She's the only person I know who wears pajamas all day—unless there's company or Sunday, always a white cotton housecoat with red flowers and pinstripe seersucker pajamas.

Another memory pops up. Grandma loves flowers. We walk through the yard to look at her giant Elephant Ear plants, deep red Calla lilies and Bleeding Hearts. Bleeding hearts have such a dainty flower, a small red heart with a white drop at the tip. It looks like the heart is bleeding or crying. She tells me how to plant flowers and how the ring of bricks helps keep out the weeds. Momma and Aunt Judy had helped her make the border with left over brick from grandpa's jobs.

We're over by the pump house, checking out her bleeding heart, and a snake crawls out from behind the plant. "It's a snake" I scream. I have only a wordless shriek to express my terror as I jump around. I grab onto Grandma for dear life. She pushes me away, grabs a hoe, and promptly chops the snake into bits.

After she calms my fears, I realize she's crying too. I think it's my fault because who would cry over a snake? "I'm sorry, Grandma. I didn't mean to make so much noise."

Hugging me close, she tells me, "You did nothing wrong. I killed it and it was just a king snake. It couldn't hurt you, baby."

She wasn't angry at me for being afraid. She was upset because she killed "one of God's creatures who couldn't do us no harm". My garden has delicate bleeding hearts in remembrance of her gentle nature.

In my thirties, I became interested in my family's history. My Aunt Vivian borrowed a book for me that traced the ancestry of my grandmother's family. According to Castles and Conquests, written by Guy Funderburk (1975), my grandmother's ancestors were minor German nobility. Around 1738, they emigrated to what was then the Carolina colony. As they approached their destination, a shipwreck killed all members of the family except Devauld. Another ship picked him up. The captain of that ship sold Devauld as an indentured servant to pay for his passage.

Funderburk also showed that the family settled in the Lancaster County, SC area. By his account, they were preachers, farmers, and merchants. Streets in Rock Hill and Fort Mill bear their names. Growing up, my family didn't talk about this, so it had no impact on my life, but it was interesting to find out later.

4

Lessons

Grandpa was a tall man. He worked as a brick mason. Some places he built in Charleston and on Johns island are still standing today. Grandpa built their brick three-bedroom house himself. Although he was the preacher in one of the small island churches, I cannot remember him talking much if he wasn't behind the pulpit.

As a child, he seemed larger than life to me. Much like historical figures appearing in biographies written for young children, I never thought he could have undesirable traits. Or being anything but "Grandpa". Like the characters in those stories, I saw him only in one dimension: Grandpa.

Even as a child, I was never a "girly girl". I spent my early childhood running around in bib overalls or a red and white cowgirl outfit, a skirt and vest with white imitation leather fringe. Just like Dale Evans on Sky King.

When Grandpa came home from work, he smelled flinty, like mortar and brick dust. First, he drank a glass of iced tea and then he got a bath. Next, we had to get through dinner. Waiting was hard. I wanted to go with Grandpa as he worked around the property. Because he left for work early, dinner was the main meal for the day. We ate about two o'clock, usually fried chicken or country fried steak with rice and gravy. Momma or an aunt brought his food to him at the big kitchen table.

After we ate, I waited on the screened-in patio with Grandma. The ceiling fan always threatened to lull me to sleep before Grandpa decided what he was doing next. If I was lucky enough to stay awake, I could help him fix the road or go fishing.

Fixing the dirt road from the state road to the house was an ongoing chore. We loaded the bed of his pale blue pickup truck with broken brick and bags of oyster shells. Grandpa drove while I hung on in the truck bed. When we got to where we were working, I'd stand up and help dump the bricks and oyster shells out in the potholes. Grandpa smashed them up a bit with a sledgehammer. Then he drove over them to pack them down.

I enjoyed working on the road, but for me, fishing with Grandpa was the best. He had a pond dredged out in the marsh. Lush, tall cattails surrounded it. After grabbing our cane poles with their red and white bobbers, we dug for earthworms in the sandy soil at the edge of a clearing. I learned to bait my hook and toss out my line. I didn't like the squirmy worms and the mess on my hands, but to fish I had to bait the hook. Once I caught the fish, I had to get it off the hook without getting a fin in my hand.

If the fish weren't biting, Grandpa shot snakes in the water. When I was around four, I decided I wanted to shoot the snakes too. Grandpa sat me on the tackle box between his knees and showed me how to line the sight up on the head of the snake and then squeeze the trigger.

Like when we fished, Grandpa made me learn all the parts of shooting; how to load the gun and how to be safe. Each time we practiced; it was the same.

"Always keep the barrel pointed at the ground when you're not shooting. Never point at something you're not shooting at. Bullets go a long way. If you're practicing, be sure your bullets can't go off and hurt someone. That's why I shoot into the water. Nothing down there but fish and snakes. Got it?"

"Yes, sir."

"Hold on tight to the gun. It's going to buck like a horse in a western. Remember to squeeze the trigger easy. Don't jerk it."

"Yes, Grandpa."

The gun was loud, but after a while I learned not to duck my head or close my eyes while pulling the trigger. His hands over mine kept the gun from flying out of my smaller ones. I caught more fish than I ever shot snakes. I learned the basics and not to be afraid of the noise.

One day Momma wanted to take a picture of me in my cowgirl outfit. I made everyone wait until I got my gun and holster. After they took the picture, everyone realized I had gotten Grandpa's loaded 38 instead of my cap pistol. Momma got upset about the revolver but eventually agreed he could keep teaching me how to shoot using his 22-caliber single-shot rifle.

Sundays were different. Everyone put on their Sunday best. Ladies wore gloves with their dresses. Even I had to give up my overalls and cowgirl skirts. I wore dresses with ruffles and sashes, white socks, and black patent leather shoes. Men wore suits and ties, if they had them, but they at least wore a shirt and tie. Grandpa gave the sermon. Momma and my aunts led the hymns. Grandpa's sermons were frightening to me as a child. It sounded to me that God had little hope for humanity, and our destiny was a fiery eternity. Sunday school was better. Beautiful pictures of Jesus talking with God as beams of sunlight streamed down from the clouds that hid God's face.

Sometimes after church there was a social, the women brought food. After we ate, the adults sat around talking and the kids ran through the churchyard trying to have fun without messing up our Sunday clothes. Across the treelined road, Black families were doing the same thing at their church, but we never joined each other. Everybody kept to their particular place. We assimilated "our place", much like we learned to talk.

When there wasn't a church social, the women of the family gathered in the kitchen and cooked dinner. Often someone outside of the immediate family was there at dinner---maybe some of the extended family or a church member and their family who were going through a rough spell. Smells of fried chicken, rice, and biscuits filled the air.

Everyone ate around the big kitchen table. After Grandpa said grace, the women prepared a plate for their spouse and children. Once everyone was served, they sat down to eat. After dinner, the men headed outside, and the women cleaned the kitchen. They tasked older children with watching after the younger ones. Sometimes, later, we had a bonfire and steamed seafood... oysters, shrimp, or crabs, whatever the family had caught earlier in the week. Grandpa held me in his lap and fed me oysters or picked out the good crab meat for me.

Before Benny was born, my parents moved our trailer from Grandpa's to behind the country store a few miles down the road. Many mornings while pretending to be asleep, I could hear Momma calling "Benny Taylor get out of that bed. Daddy will be here any minute. Come on, you gotta go to work." My dad smoked cigarettes and drank beer. Grandpa did not approve of these activities. Not long after, they sold the trailer and moved into Charleston. My dad had a new job. We visited everyone on Johns Island often, but it was not the same. Grandma was getting sicker.

Later, through family members, I learned my grandpa was not so one dimensional. His father was a member of the Catawba tribe. Family oral history says he was both Catawba and Cherokee. Maybe great-grandpa's family had joined with a Cherokee tribe. It was fairly common for small remnants of different tribes in the southeast to band together after smallpox and the federal government's efforts to make way for settlers decimated their numbers.

The Catawba's were farmers and hunters. The women produced beautiful pottery and baskets. Grandpa helped his father plow the fields with a mule and spent little time in school. His father was a hard man and Grandpa left home at a young age.

Grandpa started out as a construction laborer. After becoming a brick mason, he started his own construction company. Going through old pictures I found one of Grandpa with a motorcycle. I couldn't believe what I saw. Momma said Grandpa, at one point, rode motorcycles and hung out in bars. He stopped riding after he was in a bar fight, and someone shot a man. Another old picture of him and my grandma showed him in a Navy uniform. Apparently, he enlisted in the US Navy in World War II. I don't know how he got from the bar to the Navy to being a preacher. He died before I could ask.

As I grew older and more cognizant of social injustices, I felt at odds with my memories of Grandpa, how we all accepted the status quo. I had to unlearn a lot of things. Things like what was a woman's place and how to live with people who appear different from you. It's better to look at the whole person, acknowledging no one is one dimensional and determine where to draw a line. It is okay to keep the good they taught us while rejecting the bad and maintain the truths we have learned. So, I cherish the good things he taught me, reject the bad and accept he was flawed, as all of us are flawed.

It's important to understand our history. We have to talk about the wrongs in our society and seek to understand how seeing some monuments and names on buildings affects others. This is especially true when the monuments represent a despicable time in our nation's history. If we wipe out references to the evils in our country's past and avoid honest discussion, we open ourselves to perpetuating and repeating wrongs done in the past.

My Dad was the Milkman

Sounds funny, doesn't it? My dad drove a milk truck for West End Dairy in Charleston. Although he would come in and out of my life for another few years, this was the last time we lived together as a family for an extended period. I know he and my mother had a tumultuous marriage. They married so young.

Dad came home with things from his truck nearing their expiration date to help stretch out the food money. Who knew your milkman could deliver milk, orange juice, bacon, and eggs? When we left Johns Island, we lived in a large two-story house on Bee Street, rented inexpensively from the dairy because parts of it were falling apart, like the tiles from the coal fireplaces in all the rooms. Overall, it was a sturdy, fun place to live.

It had a big backyard with iris beds and screened in back porches. Sometimes Dad and I played wiffle ball. Of course, at five, I couldn't hit a lick, but Dad could. He showed me how to hit and we played catch. He played baseball on a company team. I remember seeing him in red pinstripes and a red baseball cap. Laughing and smiling from the dugout. Interesting, the man I never actually knew introduced me to one of my greatest passions, baseball.

And trains. For Christmas one year before I started school, I received a train set. Not the oversized ones for kids, but small ones. Dad helped me set up the track and run the trains. Side by side on the floor, we watched the train go around the track. He talked about places he had been.

Those were the good times. Most other times, I tried to make myself small and hide away from their angry shouting. I remember coming home after being out with Grandpa. Momma and my dad were sitting on the couch. It was Early American with wooden arms and wagon wheels on the side. One arm angles away from the couch. It's broken. The air is so thick with unspoken anger and pain. Momma, still in the white blouse and black skirt she wore to work, tries to get up. Dad pulls her back down to the couch. He puts his arm around her shoulder to pull her close. She can't get up. He smiles at Grandpa and me. Blood runs down her face, her neck and onto her white blouse. I run crying to Momma. Grandpa grabs me before I can get to her and sends me upstairs. I curl up on my bed with a doll and a book. More angry voices. After a while, my grandpa comes to tell me goodbye. A bit later, I hear Momma in the bathroom and then her bedroom. Then her footsteps fade away as she goes back downstairs. When she calls me downstairs, my dad isn't there. We're quiet as we eat supper. *We never talked about this incident until I brought it up to Momma when I was questioning some of my childhood memories.*

Although it took several more years, once he and my mother separated, I saw him rarely. I remember more than once waiting all day for someone who never came. When I was eight or nine, for a few weeks we stayed with Dad and the woman who became his second wife. She had a son about my age, and we played throughout the neighborhood.

The visit ended following a car accident, which left her unable to walk for a time. She had braced herself to keep my youngest brother safe. Her injuries healed without having long-term effects. My sister has two scars above one eye to this day from her head hitting the hinge on the front seat. After the accident, he was out of my life for many years.

Fragments

I've been going through family pictures. I remember eagerly waiting for Momma to share the stories that go along with the pictures. Listening intently, I try to burn the stories into my brain, never to forget. My grandfather holding year old me off the hot sand at the Isle of Palms. Another of Uncle Butch and Aunt Judy when they came to visit us in Charlotte. Now that Momma's gone, the pictures spark other memories not captured on film. They're not full-fledged stories, just fragments that hold together my feelings of family and the beach.

My sister Terry was a baby when we lived on the Isle of Palms. Back then, there were just a few houses, a small boardwalk with a carousel, restaurants, bars, and a souvenir shop. The homes were all middle class and spread out. Our apartment was right on the beach. A small picket fence separated the yard from the public beach. Momma would push Terry's stroller on the packed sand while I darted around like a sandpiper finding shells, sand dollars and other bits washed up by the tide. To me, it was perfect.

In late summer, meteorologists predicted a hurricane would hit up the coast from us. Momma sent Terry and me to stay with Aunt Judy and Uncle Butch at Grandpa's. She was volunteering at the shelter set up for those displaced by the hurricane. As hurricanes do, this one shifted. Listening to the radio, my aunt and uncle decide we should leave Johns Island. After quickly boarding up the house with plywood, they load us into Uncle Butch's car.

An eerie silence hangs in the air, which is usually filled with a cacophony of bird calls, croaking frogs, and buzzing insects. It seems as if we were the only living things around. Uncle Butch is driving unusually fast down the dirt road. The trees and bushes make a green tunnel topped by an angry slate gray sky. I look out the back window at the churning water rushing toward the car.

"Look, Aunt Judy, the beach is coming."

"It'll be okay, sugar. We'll be on the main road soon."

I keep looking back, watching the water race up the road. The car lurches to a stop. Uncle Butch leaves the motor running as he jumps out and runs to the front of the car. Aunt Judy puts Terry beside me and hurries to Uncle Butch.

"Play with Terry. Don't let her in the front seat."

With Terry behind me, I crane forward to see over the front seat and out the windshield. There's a tree down. It's blocking the road. The water is getting closer. Somehow, Uncle Butch and Aunt Judy get the tree off to the side of the road.

They scramble back into the car. Aunt Judy reaches over the seat to grab Terry. Uncle Butch puts the car in gear and hits the gas. Branches from the fallen tree scrape at the car's sides as if to hold us back. Just ahead of the water, we made it to the main road. Funny, I don't remember where we spent the night. Probably with some of our family who lived inland, I'm sure.

After the hurricane passed, Momma and I walk the beach. So many shells left stranded. The best whole conch shells I'd ever seen. Momma told me about the jellyfish and other sea creatures the hurricane had washed up on the shore.

When the younger kids were babies and sleeping, Momma and I had tea parties. I had a china tea set. Yellow and white with wheat leaves on the sides. I would set up our places with a cookie or two on our plates. Momma made instant coffee and poured it into the tiny teapot.

I filled the sugar bowl. The creamer held Carnation's evaporated milk. Momma poured. My cup held milk with just enough coffee to color it and a bit of sugar.

Another time, during winter, we three kids stayed with Aunt Judy on Johns Island. It snowed, just a flurry. We had never seen snow before, except in a book. We ran outside laughing, twirling around trying to catch the snowflakes on our tongues. When we got dizzy and tired, we helped Aunt Judy scrap snow off every flat surface into a pot. As we warmed up, Aunt Judy mixed the snow with evaporated milk and sugar. She put it in the freezer. After supper, we had snow cream.

When I was eight or nine, I stayed with Grandpa for a couple of weeks during the summer. One Saturday afternoon, Uncle Butch changed into slacks and a short-sleeved dress shirt.

"Come on, girl. Get cleaned up. Let's go skating."

Dutifully, he tried to teach me how to skate, with little success. He sat me up at a table near the rink and got us a soda and some peanuts. After sitting with me a bit, he skated with some young women his own age.

Years later, I told him how much that meant to me. "Aw, having a kid along was the best to meet the girls." Typical Uncle Butch, always self-effacing and with a heart of gold.

I don't remember my great grandma Lily. She died when I was a year old. Still, Momma's stories of her strength and determination had a considerable influence on me. At 37, Great grandma became a widow with three teenagers and two children under six. Unusual for the time, she never remarried, but continued working the farm with the help of her children. The boys, as they grew older, also worked in the mills.

Momma developed asthma as a young child. She often had further complications since they didn't have money for doctors. They only went to the doctor if you had something serious, like diabetes or tuberculosis. Anything else they treated at home. Since everyone was working, Grandma took Momma to Great-grandma Lily's when she was ill.

From her pictures, at least later in life, Great grandma was a large buxom woman. She kept her long hair arranged in a neat bun. Momma often told me how Great grandma would undo her bun each night, comb her hair 100 strokes and then braid it before going to bed. In the morning, Great grandma undid her braid, combed 100 strokes, and put her hair back in its bun. Momma never braided her hair but wore it in a neat bun until well into her thirties.

Great-grandma Lily taught Momma how to garden, can, cook and keep house. Momma often spoke of her great-grandma's strict discipline and iron will, but she also told of her kind heart. Great-grandma Lily would be among the first to help a neighbor in need. She also taught Momma to quilt, sew, and embroider. Skills Momma would later pass on to me.

Storm Clouds

Dad left West End Dairy, and we left Bee Street before I started school. We moved to a ground-floor apartment. Momma, my aunt Judy, Terry, Benny, and I lived in the one-bedroom apartment. The walls were a dark avocado green and no matter how much Momma cleaned; it smelled musty and old. Dad's absences were getting longer. Momma's bed was in the living room. I slept on a small couch at the foot of Momma's bed. Aunt Judy shared the bedroom with Terry and Benny. There wasn't much room with two cribs in there.

Not long after we moved, Momma and I walked in the scorching sun to the Health Department. I was to get my smallpox vaccination for school. I was hot, tired, and sticky. Fussing because Momma had made me wear a dress and my Mary Janes instead of shorts and tennis shoes, I pulled at her arm, trying to slow her down.

"It's so hot. Why do I have to wear this dress?"

"You don't wear shorts to see the doctor," she said.

"Why do I have to get a shot? Why can't we go to the park?"

"So, you don't get diseases, like smallpox or whooping cough."

"What's that?"

"People and especially children used to die from these diseases, but vaccinations keep them from getting the disease."

Entering school was a revelation. More books than I had ever seen. Maps. The smell of chalk. Playgrounds and tree lined parks seen from the classroom window. Ms. Wilson was tall, slender, and her curly short white hair was always neat. She could be stern, but when she first looked over her glasses; her expression made her look as if she was about to smile.

Ms. Wilson divided the class based on our ability to read. With Grandma and Momma's help, I had been reading since I was four. These were the days of Dick and Jane stories where Mother stayed home, and Father went to work each day. Not much of a challenge for one who cut her reading teeth on the *Bible*, "The Reader's Digest" and *Robinson Caruso*. Ms. Wilson talked with Momma and arranged for me to stay after school so she could teach me at my level. Aunt Judy usually walked me to and from school. We had to be home in time for Momma to go to work. Momma somehow found the money, so I could take a cab home from school.

Wayne was born while we lived there. He was so tiny when he came home. His diapers were the size of a washcloth. At first, he slept in a car basinet on Momma's bed. Momma washed him twice a day with PhisoHex soap to prevent infection. We were so afraid he would get sick. They later stopped using PhisoHex because it could affect a child's nervous system.

Dad was back. We moved to a larger upstairs apartment. It had a long balcony where Wayne could be out in the sun. Aunt Judy moved back to John's Island. With its arm propped up, that old couch with the wagon wheel arms sat in the living room. I felt sick to my stomach if I sat on it. I tried not to look at it.

If first grade was a revelation, second grade was culture shock. Momma enrolled me in a Catholic school so she could walk me to and from school and still get to work on time. Everything was completely foreign to me. We prayed and sang gospel in my church, but the concept of saying a Hail Mary was beyond my understanding. *Why are we pray-ing to Jesus' mother? Isn't it a sin to pray to anyone but God or Jesus? Why confess to a priest? Only Jesus could forgive your sins.*

Boys and girls had separate playgrounds at recess, even though we were in the same classroom for lessons. Boys played kick ball and girls jumped rope. The nuns were always on patrol; the wind catching their habits like black sails. It's also the first time I felt I didn't belong—a feeling that persisted for much of my life.

Nothing had ever prepared me for nuns---especially Sister Mary Meadows. She was a tall, slender woman who wore the traditional white wimple and black habit which reached to the top of her shoes. Sister walked up and down the rows of seats, tapping her hand with a ruler. If a child misbehaved or gave a wrong answer, she hit their hand with the ruler. Tap, tap, tap went her ruler. Tap, tap, tap went her shoes on the wooden floor. Like all good Southern children, I said yes ma'am to my female elders. After countless whacks on the palm and many silent tears, I learned to say, "Yes, Sister."

This, unfortunately, was not the worst of my transgressions. Once free from Grandpa's strict rules, Momma enjoyed wearing red lipstick and nail polish. Like many young girls, I would play dress-up with my mother's nail polish and jewelry. On one occasion, Momma didn't get all the polish off my nails. At school the next day, Sister Meadows was walking between the rows. Tap, tap, tap went her shoes. The tapping stopped at my desk. Sister grabbed my hand, squeezing hard until my fingers were white against the bright red polish. "What is this?" as she turned my hand over and struck it with her ruler.

"I was playing with Momma's nail polish. I'm sorry. I didn't get it off." I didn't understand what I had done wrong. I knew I was too young to wear nail polish except in play. I didn't do it on purpose.

"Red is for harlots. How could your mother let you do this?" Blows from the ruler accompanied her words. I stopped trying to explain as large tears rolled down my cheeks. I took a note home to Momma.

After Momma met with Mother Superior, there were no more religion classes. I sat outside of Mother Superior's office completing an assignment while my classmates studied religion. We prayed together before lunch. I was to be praying "in the manner of my faith" but I stared at her rosary. It was the most beautiful piece of jewelry I had ever seen. Tiny silver loops linked shiny black stones. All connected to a large silver crucifix. It was rather ornate compared to the crosses I saw my grandma and aunts wear. I asked how I could get a necklace like hers. To her credit, Mother Superior didn't chastise me for equating the rosary with simple jewelry but explained how it helped her say her prayers.

On Momma's days off, we often walked all over Charleston's public gardens. We saw camelias and azaleas in all shades of pink, red, and white. We were like ducks. Momma pushing the stroller with both boys in it. Terry held onto Momma, and I gripped Terry's free hand. The best times were when we could get to Johns Island. After visiting family, Momma would pack a simple picnic lunch and we'd go to the Angel Oak. Even then, the live oak branches reached to the ground and back up to the sky. The tree's vast canopy gave wonderful shade from the blistering sun. A perfect place for climbing and walking along the branches.

My parents were always trying to find a better-paying job. We moved to Rock Hill and then later to Charlotte during the school year; three schools in one year. Bruns Avenue was the street we lived on first. I liked the house; it had a plum tree in the backyard. My brothers and sister played in the yard, and I read. It smelled clean. Momma bought a red sectional sofa and kitchen table from the Salvation Army. We four kids shared one bedroom. Momma and Aunt Judy had the other.

Aunt Judy was living with us again while Momma was trying to set herself up as the manager of a diner in Cramerton. Here I discovered school libraries and checked out as many books as I could. I devoured every biography, William Penn, Lou Gehrig, Abraham Lincoln, and Elizabeth Blackwell. Sometimes, Dad came by with money for groceries. If he didn't, we ate potted meat sandwiches until Momma came home on the weekends. She'd fry chicken, give Judy money for groceries, and take us for walks to the school playground.

We moved from the house to a duplex up the street, next to Aunt Judy and her new husband. One day, my friend and I were making Fizzes in the galley kitchen. My dress caught fire as I got too close to the old-fashioned hot water heater whose burner was a few feet above the floor.

I twirled around, screaming. "Help! Help! I'm on fire! My dress is burning!"

Aunt Judy rushed into the kitchen crying, "Be still. Let me get at it." She beat the flames with her bare hands, then wrapped me in a bedspread to smother all the flames.

Aunt Judy got second-degree burns on her hands and forearms, beating out the flames. Because my nylon crinoline and tights melted to my skin, I had second and third-degree burns on my left hip. A case of chicken pox complicated the wound's healing. I had a lumpy purple and white scar on that hip well into my thirties. I did worksheets at home and completed the school year. Aunt Judy and her husband moved to West Virginia, near his family.

7

Tempest

By the third grade, we had moved again—to Cramerton. Momma was managing a diner in town. I never enjoyed living there. The apartment had a living room, one enormous bedroom with three beds, and a kitchen with a two-burner hotplate. Each apartment had a private bathroom but, you walked down a wide shared hallway to get to your toilet and shower.

The town was so small, all twelve grades were in one three story building. Sawdust on the hardwood floors was slippery. I was always afraid of falling. The "Weekly Reader" gave me some insight into the outside world. Inspired by these stories, I was going to join the Peace Corps. I would see another country and help people who were a lot worse off than I was.

When the principal called Ms. Apple to the office over the loudspeaker, I was struggling with cursive. She returned with tears running down her face and told us, "They've killed President Kennedy". I watched his funeral on a neighbor's television. I cried for Jackie and her small children. I cried about our country's loss. President Kennedy was the first living president to enter my awareness. I thought he must be a great man. Later, I would learn he was human, like the rest of us. The clouds swirling over the country following President Kennedy's death--- Vietnam, marches, riots---mirrored those happening in my personal life.

Not long after President Kennedy's assassination, we were back in Charlotte. For once, we stayed put a while or at least in the same city. My home life was unpredictable. I helped Momma with my siblings. We all had chores. Most of the time, life was peaceful. We would watch television or play board games. When we left Cramerton in the spring of 1964 and returned to Charlotte, a malevolent presence followed us. Momma remarried not long after our return. At first it was all good family fun, camping and planting a vegetable garden in the backyard.

Momma took all four of us to get our polio vaccines at school. I had a million questions about polio. She patiently told me about a childhood friend who caught polio and died. Another friend wore leg braces for the rest of his life. She brought home old copies of magazines and I read about the people in iron lungs. The clouds in my life were gathering on the horizon and threatening a hurricane.

By the time I entered junior high, he charged me with reading The Farmers' Almanac, pamphlets from the Department of Agriculture and writing reports about planting, food preservation and animal husbandry. He would grill us for hours on the breeds of various farm animals. Often, he woke us up to listen to his diatribes about the fall of modern civilization. He punished all four of us for any minor infraction, no matter who was at fault. When Momma was working, he would reduce our dinner portions, if everything wasn't perfectly in place. My stepfather was a survivalist.

I learned not to let my feelings show or cry in front of other people. *Don't give them the satisfaction of knowing they hurt you was my motto.* Futile, but it was the only rebellion I could muster. During all this, I earned money babysitting or mowing grass with the help of my siblings. Then he cut us off from our South Carolina family. Thinking about it in later years, it was as if he had read everything ever written about cults and how to break the human spirit.

The world was also changing as I entered junior high and high school. A gunman assassinated Martin Luther King. Charlotte was under a court order to integrate its schools. The school board leased older buses from the transit system, so at least the seats were comfortable and there was air conditioning.

The sense of being different, which started in the second grade, continued. I studied hard and got good grades. I was tall and loved to wear dark green. This led less kind children to call me the Jolly Green Giant. My mother worked. She had divorced my father and remarried. But half the time, my stepfather wasn't around. We didn't fit the social norms. My answer was to delve into the Russian classics, *War and Peace, Anna Karenina* and ignore my classmates.

I did well in school, mostly A's and B's. Math, except geometry, was my weakest subject, but I earned nothing less than a C. Anything else would have been unacceptable to Momma. Sedgefield's student body and its teaching staff was a conglomerate of the city. Socially conscious, my teachers held frequent sessions where they us encouraged to talk amongst ourselves about current events. They helped us see the parallels in our lives and how we all shared similar hopes and dreams. We frequently discussed the ideas of Martin Luther King, Jr., and Malcolm X. Literature classes, included the works of James Baldwin and Maya Angelou.

The Vietnam war was raging, and people were condemning US soldiers for their part in the war. I supported the soldiers but condemned the government for its policies and the draft. It was not a popular decision. They inducted me into the Honor Society for the first time. Momma smiled proudly from the audience.

The South inoculated me with racial prejudices through osmosis. By the time I finished junior high, I realized black people were just people. Their treatment should not differ from mine. It would take many years to understand how complicated implementing such a simple premise would be. No, I still don't understand why it has to be so hard.

High school found me traveling to Myers Park by bus. Talk about a fish out of water. I was now going to school with the children of college professors, city leaders, and high-level lawyers. My guard was always up, trying not to let them know how different my life was from theirs.

I worked at Eckerd's, first behind the lunch counter and then at the register. My classmates talked of working in their dad's law office, filing papers and meeting judges. All my classes were advanced placement college prep. I had no clue how I would get there, but I was determined to fulfill Momma's dream. I would go to college.

Myers Park High School looked like a small college campus. A large quadrangle edged with trees sat between the two main buildings. There were two student unions, one smoking and one nonsmoking. Students hung out on the quad during lunch, playing frisbee, talking politics, reading, or napping. Here I started listening to Elton John on a transistor radio and learned to smoke, at first sharing my friend's unfiltered Camels she swiped from her grandmother. Because of Melony, I was on the fringe of the cool kids and had a window into a hugely different world, but I didn't know how to get through the nearby door.

Unexpectedly, a door appeared. The retired Chief Petty Officer from the Junior Reserve Officer Training Corps (JROTC) came to talk to my gym class. "Women are going into new fields. The Captain and I would like to have an all-girls fancy drill team as part of our JROTC. You'll get a gym credit for participating." He explained other benefits of JROTC, but I didn't care about that. Or so I thought.

I never liked gym class. I was uncoordinated. I hated changing and showering in front of the other girls. Although developing, I was tall and gangly. They were shorter and curvier. All the whispering and giggling. Momma signed my permission slip. I loved it. I could keep in step and do complex rifle maneuvers like the Queen Anne Salute. I and a few other girls later joined the JROTC classes.

I spent little time in the library unless I was working on a paper. The reading list for my literature classes was long. It introduced to the worlds of John Steinbeck, William Faulkner, Sylvia Plath, Ernest Hemingway, and many others. I loved Faulkner's stream of consciousness. It was comforting to think others might have the same internal dialogue going on in their head while going about their daily lives. My dialogue was not the voices as described by people with schizophrenia. Rather me convincing myself to keep going, trying to make sense of the world and figure out an escape. Hemingway's conciseness fascinated me. I began writing adolescent short stories.

8

The Hurricane Makes Landfall

The hurricane hit full force when he pulled us all out of Charlotte and tossed us down in the mountains of North Carolina near the end of the school year in 1971. A three-room shack with a loft huddled in a narrow triangular valley. Cracks had formed between the rough, wide planks as they dried out. Nothing finished the inside walls. There were two outbuildings. A creek ran 300 yards from the house along one side and a natural spring bubbled out of a rocky hillside on the other. The nearest home was three miles away, along a dirt road.

The main room had a fireplace. The house had a few windows, but without paint on the walls, the inside was always dark. Each room was lit by a single bare bulb hanging from a wire in the ceiling. There were a few wall outlets, but there wasn't a 220 outlet in the kitchen. Momma and I cooked on a four-burner kerosene stove. A metal box with a thermometer served as an oven. Momma's biscuits still came out great.

No running water. We carried it up from the spring to the house daily in 5-gallon collapsible containers used for camping. Eventually, a pipe imbedded into the rock made it easier to get water into the container. No plumbing, a tent served as our bathroom. Water for bathing was heated inside and carried to the tent. After washing up at a basin, we rinsed with cold water from an improvised shower. We did laundry once a week at a laundromat.

He dropped us in this place and tasked us with planting a multi-acre garden with nothing but hand tools. Still without power tools, we four kids built a hog pen and chicken coop with rough planks we salvaged from a nearby abandoned sawmill. We cut firewood with an axe and bow saw. Eventually, he added a pair of goats to the menagerie. Every day, we staked them out and returned them to a smaller outbuilding for the night. The billy goat was mean and stinky. At least they helped keep all the brush down.

In the evening, Momma and I made curtains from feed sacks. We hung them with twine and a couple of nails. They weren't high fashion, but the curtains blocked the wind and made the cabin seem less barren, a little homier. She started teaching me how to make rag rugs like Great-grandma Lily. We didn't finish any, though.

Momma was continually working; if she didn't have shifts at the diner, she and the younger kids worked in the tobacco fields. I had a job at a takeout BBQ restaurant in a nearby town. I gave Momma whatever I earned. Supposedly, he sold real estate. Maybe he did, but Momma always paid for groceries and everything else.

There were so many snakes! I typically wore a holster with a loaded 22 caliber revolver and kept a loaded shotgun nearby to shoot the snakes. We had no way to get help if a snake bit someone. I shot them all except the black snakes. They kept the mice down. Also, I had just read Truman Capote's *In Cold Blood* and admittedly was feeling vulnerable spending so much time in the valley with just my siblings and no phone.

I was working behind the house as kids came tearing down the hill. "There are men on horses coming down the drive! Sherry!" they all called out.

"Okay, you guys go in the house and be quiet." They didn't listen, but walked through the house and stood on the front porch.

I picked up the nearby shot gun and draped it over my right arm, holding on to the trigger guard. When I made my way around the house, the two men pulled their horses up in the front yard. Dressed for riding in the country, they wore cowboy hats, jeans, and boots.

There were rifles in the scabbards of their saddles. The tallest one did all the talking.

"Well, hello ma'am." They smile, acting all friendly.

"Hi. What are you doing here? This is private property."

"Well, Hall said we could ride his land."

"This land doesn't belong to him, so go back the way you came." I shifted my shot gun which raised the barrel a bit.

Tall One dropped his reins and raised his hands near his waist, palms up. "Didn't mean to upset you none. We'll head back."

I watched them ride off. When they were out of sight, I started back to the house and made it to the front steps before my knees buckled. I managed not to throw up or cry as I took deep, gulping breaths. *If I cry, they'll all start.*

I sat on the steps as the kids gathered around. I had no illusions that my fierceness had sent them on their way; it was the sight of a nervous 16-year-old fingering the trigger on a double-barrel shotgun. Obviously, they were merely out riding, but there wasn't much I trusted in the world then. I watched the driveway and the tree line for a long time.

The yield from the garden fed us all summer and into the winter as Momma and I had canned what we didn't eat. One day I had to butcher, pluck and cook a chicken for dinner. I wasn't strong enough to wring its neck. I had to chop its head off with a hatchet. *Even as I write this, I can smell those wet chicken feathers.* I couldn't eat it. I couldn't get the smell of blood and wet chicken feathers out of my nose. For once Momma didn't scold me for not cleaning my plate and quietly gave my chicken to Benny.

Here, school was not a haven. Compared to Myers Park, everything was so parochial. We did civil defense drills sitting under our desks until the "all clear" buzzer sounded. Afterwards we watched WWII public safety movies about the dangers of radiation. English class focused more on grammar than literature.

It's getting colder. Momma and we four kids fill the cracks with more mud and paper. I haven't been to work for a week. I don't know where he is. Momma avoids talking about it, if we ask. We move more wood down to the porch. Then, seemingly out of nowhere, my Uncle Butch and his friend arrive with a car and a pickup truck. After hugging us all really tight, Uncle Butch hands us bags to shove our stuff in. Uncle Butch's friend is on the porch, pacing and watching the driveway, urging us to hurry.

"Come on now. We gotta get going. When's he coming back?"

"I don't know. We're nearly ready." Momma calls up the stairs. "Hurry kids."

In the end, all we load into the truck are bags of clothes, the remaining canned food, and the guns. The adults want to get on the road as fast as possible. It would be hard to pass anyone on the narrow driveway to the main road.

Hours later, we are back on Johns Island. We stay with Uncle Butch and his wife, Carrie. I'm free. My family is safe. I am home near the ocean. We stay there for a short while, just long enough to enroll in a school and think I might like it.

9

Storm Surge

Poof, we were back in Charlotte. No house this time, but a two-bedroom apartment. We girls had one, and the boys had the other. Momma turned the dining room into her bedroom. At least I was back at Myers Park. Now, I understood; Momma was pregnant. In those days, women lost their job when they became pregnant. Forget about getting hired while you were pregnant. No job. No money. At sixteen, I had a baby brother.

When Martin was about nine months old, Momma was in the hospital. I was terrified. I thought she might die. We rarely saw a doctor. Momma cured everything with aspirin, Vicks vapor rub, diluted Mercurochrome throat sprays or a mustard plaster.

After Terry and I cleaned up the kitchen, I prepared Martin's next bottle, just in case. At twelve, Terry knew what to do, but I was trying to make things easier for her. I worried our stepfather would come by and harass them while I was gone. There was nothing to be done, though. He had told us that Momma would be home in a few days, but I had to see her for myself.

Once I changed back into the dress I wore to school, I made my way to the hospital on buses. Following the rules on my first visit, I asked for Momma's room number at the information desk.

"What room is Mrs. Davis in?"

"Mrs. Davis is in room 304. But visiting hours are over. You need to come back tomorrow." Almost immediately, she resumed her conversation with the security guard.

Shoulders drooping, I turn to leave. As I reach the entrance door, I decide to see Momma tonight. *Who cares about their rules?* Straightening my shoulders, I drift over to a chair and pull out my bus schedule. *When's the last bus to get me home?*

Getting off the elevator, a pungent smell of disinfectant permeates the air. I notice the nurses at the station well up the hall from Momma's room. They all seem busy and don't notice me. Quickly, I follow the signs to Momma's room, afraid my shoes clicking on the tile floor would alert the nurses to my presence. I slip inside the door or her room.

Momma smiles when she sees me. "How did you get here?" Her voice is weak, and she looks sleepy.

"On the bus."

"Are the kids okay?"

"They're fine. I fixed dinner; we ate before I left. We just want you to get well and come home."

"I'll be home in a few more days. It'll be okay."

The next few days were an ordeal. I kept the house neat, cared for Martin and my other siblings. I missed about a week of school. Taking Martin with me on the bus, I collected assignments for the time I would be out of school. Keeping up with my schoolwork on top of everything else was difficult. Eventually, Momma came home. Spring turned to summer.

That summer was so long. I worked, kept house, and watched the kids while Momma worked. It was humiliating when people assumed Martin was my child as I carried him while going about my errands. I might be poor, but I was not an unwed mother. It was getting harder to remain within the eye of the hurricane. Momma didn't sing much these days. Attempting to achieve perfection was exhausting and impossible. His demands became more intense.

"Who changed the radio dial? You don't touch it. Your rooms are a mess."

He put the radio in the trunk of his car. He emptied our dressers and closets, expecting the clothes to be put back before Momma came home from work.

After my experience with the hospital and the horseback riders, I imagine was getting sassy, refusing to take the tensions at home quietly. He and Momma took me to a doctor who didn't listen to me or Momma. In those days, it was common for a doctor to listen to the male present rather than the female patient, even if the woman was of age.

"She's moody. Either crying or talking back all the time." My stepfather said.

"She's a good girl. She just---"

The doctor cut Momma off. Typical for the time, the doctor decided I was "another nervous female undergoing the throes of puberty" and put me on Librium, an antianxiety pill. Unfortunately, even today, some doctors prescribe a pill rather than seek the root cause for a woman's symptoms.

September brought the beginning of school. Things started out well. The retired captain and chief petty officer in charge of the JROTC unit convinced me I should apply to the US Naval Academy when it opened enrollment to women.

We girls in the JROTC unit had our own drill team. We had learned all the fancy drill maneuvers like Queen Anne's salute. I don't remember why, but we couldn't compete in the annual citywide drill competition at the Charlotte Coliseum. Still, we put on an exhibition. Everyone said we did really well.

The unit had a military ball in the winter. The first dance at was to be a traditional waltz. With help, I taught the guys in the unit how to waltz. To this day, if not thinking, I will lead during a slow dance. A friend from the unit was my date for the evening. I wore an emerald green velvet formal. With its empire waist bodice and bell-shaped sleeves trimmed with gold braid, I felt like a renaissance princess.

In the spring, there were riots at school. Someone bludgeoned a student to death in a school parking lot. Some people said he had a gun and threatened another student. Others said outside agitators, not students, attacked him. I don't think they ever found out exactly what happened.

After this, police officers were everywhere in the school, every building entrance, every hallway intersection, along the walks between buildings. The school board suspended extra-curricular activities. Students could no longer gather on the quad. Extra police officers stood near the protracted line of buses at the beginning and end of each school day and in the student and teacher parking lots. Lockdowns became commonplace.

While I don't condone violence, I can understand the frustration of many black people. Children, mostly black, from less affluent neighborhoods, endured the hassles of traveling to and from school on buses. The courts approved the redistricting plan for schools. However, few students from affluent neighborhoods traveled across town to go to school.

It became apparent the US Navy would not allow women to enter the Naval Academy by the time I would graduate. The first female cadets didn't enter until 1976. That door closed, but is there another?

A teacher, whose husband was a professor at Queens College, told me about a scholarship program for high school students. The student enrolled in their senior year. It was a full scholarship. I could work on campus to earn spending money. I just needed to get the financial aid paperwork completed. Momma thought it was a good idea. He said no. Later he changed his mind, but said I would have to live at home.

For me, this was the last straw. I started planning. It took a couple of months for me to squirrel away enough money and find a place to live. In the early 70s, women didn't have bank accounts of their own. Besides, I was a minor. Chief let me lock my money in his desk drawer. I felt guilty; until now, I always gave Momma whatever money I had left after buying clothes and school supplies, but I knew I couldn't continue this way.

This phase of my life ended with a few tears, but no fanfare. I moved into the maid's studio apartment in a classmate's home. It had a small kitchen and a bathroom. I rented that room for a few months until her parents found the roach clip left there by their daughter. Of course, I had to move. They didn't believe her when she told them she smoked there while I was at work.

I rented a room from Melony's brother- and sister-in-law. I worked. I kept going to school. Melony and I often sat in Waffle House drinking coffee and writing bits of stories on napkins. We talked about the expatriates we studied in lit class and how we would grow up to be tragically famous like they were. I did stupid teenaged things like get drunk with my girlfriends. Usually, we hung out in my room while drinking. Of course, the drinking age was eighteen then.

During one lockdown at school, I talked with Chief about not being able to go to college. "You could enlist in the Navy. The GI Bill pays for college once your enlistment is up," he offered.

"I'm not sure about going so far away."

"You don't have to decide today. Think about it. Boot camp won't be easy. The Navy won't be easy either, but you could do it."

After thinking for a short time, I talked with Momma. I decided to enlist. Chief gave me a ride to the recruiting center. I had credit for 3 years of JROTC. I would be an E-3 after completing boot camp. They delayed my enlistment for a month because, as a young woman, I needed parental permission to enlist since I was under twenty-one.

I stopped by the apartment to say goodbye the day before flying out to Orlando. We visited and ate the snacks I brought with me. I caught Momma up on my program. I was to go to San Diego to train as a dental technician once was boot camp was over. It was indescribably hard to leave my family, the pain, the guilt. Even now, there are no words to encompass everything I felt. I didn't know how they would survive or what was ahead of me. I just knew I had to do it. Too soon, my ride was at the door. After a last round of hugs for everyone, pale faced and crying, I walked through the door to my tomorrow.

This time of my life was not all terrible. He wasn't around for days at a time. When it was just the Momma and we five kids, we played gin rummy, canasta and parchesi. One Halloween, we dressed up in home-made costumes and bobbed for apples because the younger kids couldn't go trick or treating. Momma taught me to embroider pillowcases and the edges of flat sheets. We even made purses out of embroidered burlap strips. It was so trendy, with orange and yellow daisies. Like all of us, he caught Momma in this Rasputin like spell. Fortunately, she eventually broke the spell for herself and my siblings.

10

Thoughts on Education

Today, school boards are discussing cutting out advanced placement classes. Often their reasoning has to do with budgets and supposed racial disparity. These classes should not require a tutor, a special class to gain entrance or fees. If they do, then the entrance requirements are wrong.

I shudder to think how different my life would have been if a teacher had not recognized my abilities. Or if advanced placement classes had not been available to me. No one in my family could have provided the knowledge gained there. Nor could they have even told me where to look to find it.

I am troubled that today's children from marginalized races and cultures might lose this important opportunity. My incessant reading showed me that there were other ways to live. Even if college is not part of your plans, what you learn from the study of literature, science and math is invaluable, as it can show you what is possible. The end goal of education, once it prepares you for making your way in the world, should teach people to think for themselves, to take in information and draw your own conclusions, not rote memorization of facts.

To be honest, there was an element of chance or luck, if you will, in the pivotal moments of my early life: integration sent me to a school in a very affluent neighborhood, much different from the one I would have originally gone to, I could find a safe place to live through friends and good teachers helped me. Yes, I worked hard, but so did many others whose circumstances denied them the same opportunity.

The attitude that you just need to "pull yourself up by your bootstraps" has prevailed in our country for a long time. Maybe that was possible many years ago. I'm not sure it's true anymore. I believe that as a society, we should ensure that everyone has the same opportunities for education, healthcare, and participation in society. In order to achieve this goal, our schools should depart from teaching to standardized testing. Education should help children learn to think, not just regurgitate facts. It should help prepare them for life by setting them up to learn a trade or profession. It should help them learn to take in information and arrive at conclusions---to think independently.

11

Fair Seas and Following Winds

My blue matching Samsonite suitcase and overnight bag sat by my bedroom door. The large suitcase held pajamas, underclothes, and toiletries purchased from the list provided by my recruiter. The overnight bag waited for the last-minute addition of things I needed before I left in the morning. Little did I know other baggage would accompany me for several decades; PTSD and bouts of depression, but that's for later.

Sleep didn't come easily. Everything Chief told me about boot camp kept running through my mind. I worried about not being able to help Momma and the kids from so far away. *What would Florida be like? I've never been outside North or South Carolina.* I fell asleep.

Mid-morning, my recruiter stopped by with two other enlistees and took us to Douglas Municipal Airport for the first leg of our flight. After a quick lunch, the recruiter handed over our orders and wished us well. There was a brief layover in Atlanta. Of course, we disembarked at the opposite end of the airport from our connecting flight. Sprinting across the airport, we boarded our plane with just a few minutes to spare. Finally, we arrived in Orlando. It was dark by the time everyone gathered and climbed onto the old buses for the ride to the base.

As the buses unloaded at the base, we split up by sex. Petty officers led us into a dimly lit, narrow concrete hall. Their voices echoed in the narrow hallway as they instructed us to turn over items from a list of contraband posted every few feet on the facing wall. Once we bagged and labeled our things, we put them in a storage area for collection once we graduated. More booming voices as they called out names and numbers.

Traversing several stairwells led us to our company area, home for several weeks. They had divided the sizeable area into eight or nine cubicles, much like many offices. Each cubicle contained three sets of bunk beds and sometimes a single bed with individual lockers for personal items. The petty officer leading us barked orders for us to stow our things by the locker assigned. Too tired for chatter, I find the locker with my name, set down my luggage and stand outside the cubicle.

"Attention on deck." At the other end of the cubicles stands a slender woman, about 5 feet tall with dark short hair. She cradles her bucket hat securely under her right arm. Her voice thunders as if from a loudspeaker.

"I am DI Maxwell. Your company commander. Each of you will have duties to maintain the cleanliness of company areas, as well as your bunk and locker. The head has a shower room and laundry room. There will be daily inspections. Do you understand?"

"Yes, ma'am." We answered, a bit ragged. We'd learn to do that loudly and in unison before long.

"Next to my office is the lounge. If the smoking lamp is lit, that is where you smoke after dark. All ashtrays are to be emptied in the red bucket. There is no smoking anywhere else in the building. Do not leave the company area without permission. Do you understand?"

"Yes, ma'am." A little more in unison this time.

"Get your bunks made and start stowing your gear. The smoking is lit until 2130. Lights out is at 2200. Reveille is at 0500. Dismissed."

"Yes, ma'am."

Reveille blasts from a speaker. Right above my head. *I got to get up and hit the line.* Next thing I know, I'm on my back, on the deck. I look up to see people clustered around me. "Are you okay?" Once they determine there were no broken bones, a petty officer escorts me to sick bay. I was x-rayed and received a cursory exam, along with Flexeril for muscle spasms and Tylenol. So much for Navy medical care. At least they reassigned me to a lower bunk.

Weeks passed quickly as they issued my work uniforms and fitted me for dress uniforms. I attended classes in Naval history and organization and received inoculations for all the diseases prevailing outside the US. Yellow fever, cholera to name a few. Unlike the health department, which used regular syringes, hospital corpsmen with air syringes spaced themselves about four feet apart. As you reached the corpsman, you received an injection and kept walking to the next corpsman, who gave you another shot. I was lucky and didn't have a reaction to any of the injections. After the medical exams, I had to give up my wire rims for ugly black frames.

There was always scuttlebutt going around. None of us really knew anything, but we acted like we did.

"Did you hear? Marcie's getting sent home. Apparently, she's got some medical condition they didn't catch before."

"No way!"

"I got demerits for having a dirty soap dish. Wet soap melts. How do you stop it?"

"Just wash in shampoo. Baby shampoo works best, and it's cheap."

The baby shampoo trick worked for a while until someone got dinged for not showering, because the imprints on the soap were fresh. That night, we all took our bars of soap to the showers and rubbed those imprints down.

We marched everywhere. To chow, to class and back. There are male recruits on the base, but the companies were not coed, and the male barracks were in a separate building. If a male company passed near us, the squad leader would give each company a command of "Eyes right or Eyes left" to avoid looking at a company of the opposite sex. Silly right? I'm not sure why this was even a rule. What did they think we can do as the two companies passed?

On Saturdays, we shopped at the Exchange in groups. Even in groups of two, we marched. I bought stationery, toiletries, and money orders to send home to Momma. I was making about $355 a month with no real expenses other than keeping my uniforms sharp. *So much money; I'm doing good now.* If you had permission to use the phone, there were banks of pay phones. The lines always snaked around the phone area and long-distance calls were expensive.

I filled my letters to Momma with naïve statements about the Navy. I would ramble on about the importance of the quartermaster's deck and other stuff I was learning. What did I know about anything? In what turned out to be a lifelong pattern, I jumped in; fully embracing all aspects of this new venture and determined to be the best. Shortly after I left Charlotte, Momma and the kids were back in South Carolina.

In some ways, boot camp was a disappointment. Chief had prepared me to expect an obstacle course, firefighting, firing range and fancy drill. None of these things happened. Of course, it had been thirty years since he was in boot camp and his experience as a man differed from that of women. Firefighting was a perfect example. Instead of entering a fire in a simulated ship's compartment and donning firefighting gear, we had two instructors light different classes of fires in cut off steel drums. They then taught us which fire extinguisher to use. Then we had to show them the proper technique, but we didn't run into a building with a controlled fire while learning shipboard firefighting techniques.

I didn't really mind not doing the firefighting, the obstacle course, or the firing range. The Navy would never station me on a ship because I wasn't a nurse. I knew I wasn't athletically strong, and I knew I could shoot. It was a matter of principle—why have different standards for men and women? I knew women didn't serve in combatant areas. Hospital ships were as close as women got to combat zones. No guns. Not even for drill. But not to use a rifle in fancy drill. That hurt. I was good at it and wanted to show off.

In boot camp, we had to adhere to behavior standards for women from the somewhere back in the 1950s. One ring. Post type earrings if you had pierced ears. Otherwise, no earrings. No panty hose. Uniform skirts came down to the crease at the back of your knee. A professional look but vastly different for those of us used to wearing miniskirts and jeans. If I wore a dress uniform, I had to wear a girdle. With stockings. By graduation we could wear pantyhose but we still had to wear the girdle.

Really, girdles? There were no overweight women in my company. Boot camp always settles out your weight. If you're overweight, you lose and if underweight you gain. When I had my pre-enlistment physical, I weighed 120 pounds. At 5'8", I had had to gain five pounds to enlist. By the end of the boot camp, I weighed 135 pounds, which was considered my ideal weight by medical professionals. No female recruit had a tummy bulge which needed reigning in to wear the A-line skirts of our dress uniforms.

Orlando in July and August was hot. Heat exhaustion was a real thing. Everywhere there were water coolers and paper cups. Company Commander handed out salt tablets daily. We learned to watch the flags flying over the command building. No PT on red flag days. No double time on black flag days.

Besides snakes, heights scare me silly. To graduate from boot camp, we had to jump from a diving board, float, and swim to the side. It's not the Olympics, so e form and style didn't matter. It's supposed to show your ability to save yourself after an accident at sea. I couldn't jump. If I went into the water from the side, I could push off/swim to the middle, float, and swim back to where I started. Every time, at the end of the diving board, I froze. Cheeks blazing red with embarrassment, I backed my way to the ladder and crept down. It didn't matter what anyone yelled or cheered. I was terrified of that jump. They sent me to remedial swim during free time. Still couldn't do it.

They set me back two weeks to a new company. I still couldn't jump off that board. *If I don't pass this round of classes, they'll send me home.* Besides my hurt pride, I worried about having to go back to Charlotte. *How would I ever get to college? How could I return to that life?* One afternoon, during swim class, an instructor called me over to the side of the pool.

"Taylor, why are you in this class? You're doing fine out there."

"I can't get off the diving board, ma'am."

"Get out and come with me."

"Yes, ma'am."

I follow her up the ladder. Sweat mingles with water from the pool that adheres to my skin and my stomach is doing flip-flops. Up on the board, she takes my hand and walks me right to the edge. The board bounces slightly as she turns to face me. The flip-flops in my stomach become more intense with each movement of the diving board. Somehow, I don't throw up.

"Take a good breath. We're jumping in a minute" and she pulls me off the board. No delay. No chance to be more scared than I already am.

As we surfaced, "You did it. Now go do it again. You got to do it yourself to graduate. Just run and go. Don't think." I did it. Finally.

Graduation was coming soon. We often wore our service dress light blues. I was so excited. I tried to buy tickets for Momma and the older kids to come to graduation, but they couldn't make it. I really missed seeing them. Anyway, I wouldn't have had time to spend with them as my orders sent me to San Diego straight away.

When I talk about the women's movement, especially as presented in the 1970s, I never embraced the concept that women should be more than men or that men were inherently flawed. I just wanted to go about my life as a fully functioning human being without someone saying, "Girls can't do that". I look forward to the day when we no longer feel compelled to make statements regarding "the female pilot or female scientist". They are just pilots or scientists. Maybe it will be so for my granddaughters.

12

San Diego and a Cold Ocean

The flight to San Diego was long but uneventful. I traveled in my dress uniform. It had the advantage of making me appear older. So, when the flight attendant offered wine with my meal, I accepted. Of course, back home, you could buy beer and wine at 18. It allowed me to relax and doze a while before landing. That's when I learned a drink made flying so much more pleasant.

Once more, I'm awakened by a voice over a microphone, but I'm not so jumpy this time. "Please place your tray tables in the upright position and fasten your seatbelts. We will begin our descent to San Diego shortly."

Despite my fear, I looked out over San Diego. From my aerial window, I could see for miles. White lights line the dark streets like diamonds on black velvet. Traffic lights shining like rubies and emeralds mark the blocks. We land; I disembark. *Now what? Get my luggage. Get a cab.* Before landing, I had slipped a few dollars in the small pocket of my skirt so I could tip the porter without opening my purse. Everyone had warned me to be careful of pickpockets. This time, there was no one to meet me.

I locate the baggage claim area and collect my luggage. People are everywhere, but no porters in sight. I spot the luggage racks. Awkwardly, I corral my luggage. To accommodate my uniforms, I now have two large suitcases and the overnight bag.

"Excuse me, ma'am. Let me give you a hand." A petty officer offers. "Where you headed."

"The Naval Training Center. I'm scheduled for 'A' school there." We settle my luggage on the rack.

"Oh, yeah. You gotta report the WAVES barracks. They'll shuttle you to class. I'm waiting for someone on another flight. But here, I've got a few minutes. Let's get you a cab."

The cab zips through the traffic of downtown San Diego. So many people are out and moving around the city. Shore Patrol stops us at the gate. After checking my ID, we continue to the barracks. Once I finish checking in and getting basic info on the chow hall and such, I spend the night in a transient room. Wow, such a letdown. I didn't expect a red carpet. However, I quickly learned in the Navy you're just a number. I'd get my regular room and duty assignment tomorrow.

The rooms were pleasant. Odd thing to say about barracks. Recently constructed, everything was orange and yellow with a few punches of green thrown in, very modern, very 70s. Four two person rooms opened on to a lounge area with a television. Each pair of rooms connected to a Jack and Jill bathroom. I didn't have a roommate. Cool. There were six of us in the group. All going to Dental Technician (DT) "A" school.

We kept a coffee pot and toaster oven in the lounge. We went in together and bought a small refrigerator. It was much better having coffee and toast in our lounge. That way, we avoided the catcalls and propositions from guys hanging out barracks windows as we walked the several blocks to the chow hall.

They held DT school in a two-story World War II building on the far side of the base from the WAVES barracks. Originally deemed temporary, it became permanent, or as military personnel describe them temporary-permanent. Tall windows, white (probably asbestos) siding and hardwood floors were typical. No central air. Asphalt surrounded the twelve buildings. No landscaping.

Dental Technician school was more relaxed than boot camp. Still, we assembled outside first thing to hear the Plan of the Day or POD. The

POD was your schedule for the day and let you know what was coming up. Who had duty and what time you had watch. You might be on duty for 24 hours, but your watch might be from 4 pm to midnight.

The uniform of the day was included because there were so many variations available: dress whites, dress light blues and a modification of the service dark blue in the summer. There are many more variations for women. There were often differences based on the service members' function. Also, each command had its own ideas about what was appropriate.

There were about fifty of us in the class, seventeen of which were women. There was a mix of ranks as well. A few petty officers, but mostly E-3's like me. Some had been to sea or had duty at another command before changing their rating.

The men's barracks for E-3's and below were a short walk from the classroom building. It was another temporary-permanent building. I was glad that the women's barracks were in a newer part of the base. Even if it meant riding in the ancient gray bus to get to class. We could have private vehicles, but few of us had the money to buy one. Besides, none of us knew what our orders would be after "A" school, so it paid to be patient and ride the bus. A few of the petty officers owned a car.

I learned dental anatomy, how to take x-rays of the mouth and pass instruments as a chair side dental assistant. After listening to lectures, we broke up into study groups unless there was a practicum. Those who did well had a better chance of landing their preferred duty station. As we learned chairside assisting, my hands started breaking out in an itchy rash. We didn't wear gloves, as we weren't working on people. Nothing I bought in the Exchange really seemed to help. I got permission to go to sick bay.

Another temporary-permanent building. Go in. Sign in. See a Corpsman who asks a few questions and then has you wait to see a doctor. See the doctor. He looked at my hands, but hardly listened to me. "So many changes for a young woman. You need to relax." I left with a prescription for valium.

My study group included a petty officer who was currently a yeoman and had done a tour off the shore of Vietnam. Jim became more solicitous as I began having difficulty focusing during the day while taking the valium. I had already cut down the number of times I was taking it.

We went out several times to the petty officers' club. It was nicer than the non-com club, where you couldn't avoid the groping and overly eager sailors. He tried to teach me to shoot pool. After a long night of talking and finding out we liked/wanted many of the same things, books, family, children, he proposes. I accept, thinking we'd be engaged for a while.

The only way to ensure our transfer to the same duty station was to choose a large command and get married before graduation. With some consternation, I agreed, even though things were moving fast. I really wanted my mother at my wedding. Jim was six years older and had more time in the Navy. In October, we married in a wedding chapel in San Diego attended by a few friends from class.

Base housing wasn't available to students. We found a furnished apartment off base. Those few months set the tone for much of our married life. Fridays and Saturdays I'd cook for friends as we drank through the afternoon and played games like Risk. Cooking was a struggle, as my repertoire held few entrees: fried chicken, spaghetti, meatloaf, and spam. Jim would occasionally jump in with steaks or hamburgers. I didn't admit to knowing about spam, but soon started buying cookbooks and experimenting. I cooked my first thanksgiving dinner there; sharing it with a few friends. The gravy came from a packet.

We also took time to see places like the San Diego Zoo. It was the first zoo I saw with animals placed in areas which simulated their natural habitat. Often, we went to the beach. There weren't as many shells or birds as I was used to seeing. Excited to dip my toes in the ocean water, I rolled up my pant legs and ran in about ankle high. And ran back out again, surprised that without a Gulf Stream, the Pacific was cold in November.

Not long after, I was up for duty at the barracks. Jim dropped me off and drove back to the apartment. Once I reported in, I found I didn't have a watch but was a supernumerary in case of an emergency. At noon, a group of us headed to the quarterdeck for muster. We were laughing on the landing when I took a long step right to the bottom.

The Petty Officer of the Day called the medics. They carted me off to the hospital. I had a few scrapes and bruises, but not much else. As expected, the doctor ordered blood work and x-rays. The doctor seemed sympathetic and did several tests, trying to determine why I stepped off the landing and had no recollection of doing it.

Then my blood work came back.

"There is no way your blood levels can be this high if you are taking the medication as prescribed."

"I don't take it every day and never over two in a day."

"Where's the bottle?"

"At home. I'm on duty. They make me sleepy so I didn't bring them."

He reaches for the phone and calls Jim to verify my story. The doctor instructs him to give the bottle to the Shore Patrol when they arrive. More waiting. An hour goes by before the doctor reenters the exam room. "Let's see what we have here" as he dumps the pills into a counter "You've got more here than I would have thought.".

"I know."

Sympathetic doctor is back. "Look, you don't seem to metabolize drugs very well. No matter who prescribes it, never take valium again. You were lucky. I'm going to put you off duty for a couple of days so you can get it out of your system. Get dressed. Your husband is in the waiting room." This is how I wound up being the only woman wearing dress dark blues in my graduation picture. I wasn't there to hear the POD for picture day.

Our orders to the dental center at Great Lakes arrived. The Navy packed and shipped our household goods to the Naval Training Center. Jim marked the route to East St. Louis in an atlas. We would stay with his parents for a couple of days and then head up to the base outside Waukegan.

Politically in the US and globally, a lot was happening. US troops had gone into Laos and Cambodia. Spiro Agnew resigned from the Vice Presidency. The Israeli's six-day war occurred, and the Organization of Oil-Producing Countries (OPEC) came into being.

Gas jumped to 55 cents a gallon as OPEC started placing embargos on countries. People were afraid they wouldn't be able to get gas. They lined up for gas. Often, the gas station would run out before the end of the line. Eventually, each state came up with a rationing system. The most common being purchasing gas on even or odd days according to the last number of your license plate.

Years later, the irony would hit me. One reason I was eager to leave Charlotte was the fear I would marry young and felt that would be a poor decision. So, what did I do? Moved across the country and married young. Still, my first marriage gave me two wonderful sons, and the Navy brought so many experiences, which added to my growth as a person.

13

Beaches??

We started the trip before sunrise. There was a lot of uncertainty about being able to find an open gas station on our route, so we had five gallons of gasoline in the trunk. The trip was a blur of southwestern countryside. I had bronchitis again. I didn't have a license and kept falling asleep since reading in the car gave me a headache. Jim had me tick off the new states he visited in the atlas. We grabbed fast-food takeout lunches. We didn't stop until long after dark at a motel along the road. Breakfast at a diner and back on the road.

As we neared Missouri, the weather changed. Sleet and snow reduced visibility. To me, the snow packed road looked ice covered. Never having seen more than an inch or two of snow, I gripped the armrest, scared we would skid off the road into a ditch before reaching his parents' house. We arrived unscathed. We stayed a couple of days before heading to Great Lakes. I never adjusted to the cold winters by Lake Michigan.

We rented a furnished house off base for a few months until our request for base housing came through. Our possessions remained in storage. The landlady was a little odd. She insisted we pull up the shades halfway each morning. If we forgot, there would be a note on the front door when we returned from work. We later found out; it had been her mother's home and her mother always raised the shades each morning when she was alive.

Occasionally, we would go to the parks near Lake Michigan. The locals called the shoreline beaches. It was sandy, but it didn't look like any beach I had ever seen. I was severely disappointed. Maybe at our next duty station, we would be near a real beach.

The dental center had three different clinics; Naval Training Center (NTC), Recruit Training Center (RTC), and a prosthetics lab, which also provided regular dental care to retired personnel. The clinic on the NTC was another two-story WWII temporary permanent building. Downstairs contained the administrative offices, conference room, the women's locker room, the area for dental cleanings, as well as a large meeting room.

I worked chairside in NTC clinic with a general dentist. We also had two oral surgeons onboard. All areas except the actual dental exam rooms had the same muddied red low nap carpeting. Old wood tinted blinds covered the windows. Chairs for patients circled the waiting area. A receptionist sat in a corner surrounded by file cabinets and an outer counter.

Each day I got the records for that day's appointments; assembled the exam kits and set the room up prior to the doctor's arrival. We saw about ten patients a day. After each patient, I cleaned the room and placed the instruments into a sanitizing soak. Before lunch, I scrubbed and sorted them into exam kits. I then put them into the autoclave for sterilization. Lunch would find several hearts or spades games in progress. I became quite good at spades. The afternoon was just a repeat of the morning.

The Navy approved our housing request. We moved into the downstairs two-bedroom apartment of a four-unit building. The Navy constructed the apartments from unpainted concrete slabs during the 1940s. They were not so affectionately known as the Flintstones. There were three units set up around a horseshoe shaped sidewalk with a large grass filled shared area inside the horseshoe. At the top of the horse-shoe was a group of four three-bedroom units. Facing us was another four unit building of two-bedroom apartments. There were a few trees and shrubs.

The apartment interiors were all the same, with black asphalt tiles throughout. It took at least two coats of wax to have them look clean. Periodically, you had to strip off the wax or else the floor looked dirty. All the walls were a bumpy, bright white. The texture was not so much design as the result of years of repainting. There was a laundry room and storage room off the kitchen. The eat-in kitchen held a small four burner gas stove. We eventually purchased a dishwasher that rolled up to the sink. All the parking was on the street.

After work and on the weekends, we furnished the apartment. I planted my first flower garden here: nasturtiums and zinnias. Eventually, life fell into a routine. We visited clubs based on the night of the week. Weekends involved drinking and eating while playing card and board games. I learned to play backgammon and cribbage.

The best part of living in the Flintstones was the community. None of us were from the same part of the country and several of the wives were from different countries, the most common being the Philippines, Japan, and Greece. We would barbeque out in front of the buildings, and everyone brought a dish to share. If someone needed help, everyone pitched in. If someone was moving out, they would host a moving/painting party where everyone would help clean and paint. I've never found that sense of community anywhere else.

Not long after moving into the Flintstones, they transferred me to the dental clinic on RTC. At first, I worked chairside. Same routine but more patients, as there was a push to have them ready before graduation. Whatever the condition of their oral health at enlistment, the goal was to eliminate anything would "blow up" while they were at sea without a dentist available.

Prior to my enlistment, no one I knew cursed. I grew up sheltered from most social interactions. I turned beet red when my male coworkers "cussed like a sailor". Not a proud moment but, I soon could throw it back at them. Swear words rolling glibly off my tongue silenced that form of harassment. Mostly I tried to ignore the dirty jokes and innuendos directed at myself and the other women. I complained about some raunchy pornography a dentist had taped to his ceiling, "It's there to distract the patients," he laughed. The head of the clinic transferred me to the Central Sterilization Room (CSR). Everyone thought it was a joke and didn't understand why I was upset.

All the work chairside and in CSR exacerbated the rash which first appeared in San Diego. Wearing gloves didn't help. When visits to sick bay didn't yield results, they referred me to dermatology at the hospital. Testing revealed my nickel allergy. Most dental instruments are nickel plated. My choices were to request work in an administrative area of the center or to apply for an honorable discharge. I remained in the Navy and began working in the Records Section of the recruit clinic. I didn't want to give up my income or my GI Bill.

From the records department, we scheduled recruits appointments in the clinic and maintained their dental records. A third-class petty officer was in charge, and I worked with two other E-3's. We set up new dental records, which would include a history and physical and blank forms for charting their dental health. All in paper. We pulled records for follow-up appointments and sent dental records forward to the Recruit Training Center for inclusion with other records upon transfer to a permanent duty station. Shortly after I made E-4, the lead Petty Officer left the Navy, and I became responsible for the records section. Jim was taking night classes to get his master's degree.

About this time, the Navy restructured its dental centers and build the long-awaited replacement for the NTC dental clinic. Instead of being a department under the auspices of the Naval training Center, the dental clinics would become their own command. This meant they would now be responsible for their own auxiliary functions, such as personnel, supply, and finance. As a married couple made up of two enlisted personnel, we were an anomaly to the command. When I was first moved to the administrative offices, Jim was my supervisor, as he was the lead Petty Officer for administrative staff. It wasn't a pleasant situation.

The Master Chief Petty Officer of the Command (MCPOC) decided he needed an assistant other than the civilian did his typing. He chose me for the role. The MCPOC advocated for enlisted personnel when they felt they had a grievance. Under his guidance and working with one civilian secretary, I set up an office with the requisite files, policy manuals, and disseminated daily message traffic. His guidance took the form of "read the manual, if you aren't sure, ask me". The experience served me well years later when I worked as a director of nursing and often updated policies or wrote new ones.

Around this time, I developed a bleeding ulcer. We didn't address how much I was drinking and smoking. No one addressed the effects of the stress of being the part of the only married couple at the command, of trying to be perfect while being harassed for being female and "taking up a shore billet" or just because. No, just a prescription for Carafate and an admonishment to avoid spicy food. I certainly didn't realize that my body was working to tell me something.

When I was twenty-one, Momma told me Dad had contacted my brothers and sister. He wanted to talk with me too, but she felt I should decide whether I wanted him to call. I said she could give him my number. We talked on the phone a few times. Jim and I took leave to go down to Charlotte for a visit, but it was hard to find common ground. Their lives revolved around church activities, and I had stopped going to church when I was a teenager. I devoured books, but books held little interest for them.

Our administrative spaces were getting crowded, particularly as officers were coming in to head the newer departments. We moved the administrative offices to a refurbished chief's barracks that became the command building. About this time, I made E-5. They assigned me to a lieutenant in charge of the personnel department. A civilian maintained the actual personnel files. I maintained policy manuals, forwarded message traffic, and conducted audits throughout the command to ensure we were ready for our annual inspection. I often created my own audits based on my knowledge of the policy manuals. Another experience I would draw on later.

Have I mentioned we drank a lot? Everything was an excuse: wetting down parties, retirement parties, transfer parties, moving out cleaning/painting parties. Oh, it's Wednesday. "Take your civies in because we can go to the Chief's club after work." Weekends meant day long drinking and potlucks. Sometimes we drank pina colada milkshakes all afternoon as we ate, played board games and cards. Risk was no longer in vogue. War games with miniature warships, and Richthofen's War, took its place.

The Navy never considered drinking an issue if you showed up for work and weren't actually drunk on duty. I worked with a Chief who called us to his office one morning to see the people dancing outside his window. The Navy sent him to rehab. Afterwards, he quietly retired. It took years for the Navy to acknowledge its drinking problem.

We spent the holidays with Jim's family. They weren't close like mine. Jim often hunted with his dad while I stayed home with his mom. After the guys dressed the meat, I'd help his mom get it ready for the freezer. We saw a lot of Cardinals baseball since his mother could get tickets from her work.

The year before he entered Officer Candidate School (OSC), Jim sold our Dodge Colt and bought a Duster. He and a friend turned it into a hot rod. They rebuilt the engine, added a four-barrel carburetor and dual exhaust. It was fast, loud, and temperamental to drive. I loved it.

The last winter we spent in Great Lakes was among the area's worst. Temperatures stayed in the teens so long stores sold T-shits with the imprint "I survived the winter of 1976". We had office pools predicting when the temperature would finally reach freezing. The snow removal crews could not keep up. Piles of snow hid roadside signs because the road crews were running out of places to dump the snow. Each night, Jim linked extension cords together and ran them from the apartment to an inline engine heater. He still had to start it every four hours and let it idle to keep its engine from freezing. Jim completed his master's degree, and the Navy accepted him for OCS in the spring. We sold the Duster and bought a Plymouth Fury.

Prior to his departure, the officers' wives invited me to several of their club meetings to help give me an idea of what the Navy expected of an officer's wife. I learned about calling cards, china and serving tea from a silver service. At the office, the Captain told me that during any functions, I was "to mill about smartly, chat a bit and move on". Jim flew out to Newport, Rhode Island, for OCS.

I completed my enlistment in July 1977. I stayed in housing since Officer Candidate School was—for obvious reasons unaccompanied duty. Not long after he left, my aunt called to tell me my youngest brother, Wayne, died in a swimming accident while my siblings were visiting my dad in Charlotte.

I flew to Momma in Virginia. The only tickets available were first class. The flight attendant kept offering drinks, and I drank them. Aunt BJ and Momma picked me up at the airport. My aunt drove us to Manassas while I tried to sober up in the backseat. The plan was for the Momma and I to drive to Charlotte early in the morning. My aunt would fly down in time for the funeral. I needn't have worried about sobering up. Momma's neighbors had brought over trays of food, so we ate and continued drinking.

Dad and his wife lived in Charlotte. We stayed in nearby Lancaster with my Aunt Judy. After a quick change, we attended the viewing. It was surreal, my baby brother in a casket. I can still see his face. Afterwards, I stopped by my dad's for a brief visit. It was a brutally raw experience. Plans for the funeral procession included two family cars. We argued about where I was staying and in which car I would ride. They felt I should ride in the same car as my dad. So, the "family" could be complete.

"What about Momma? You have Frances' children, Terry, and Benny. She has only her sisters and brother. She needs to have at least one of her children with her."

"We want to get to know you better and come together as a family."

While I could understand their position, I rode with Momma. This set the tone for my relationship with my dad. We never became close.

When I returned to Great Lakes, it was time to get ready for the movers. I packed what I wanted to take with me. I would go first to East St. Louis, then to Manassas to see Momma, and finally to Newport. The movers made quick work of packing and were soon on their way. I sold the dishwasher, washer and dryer and their new owners picked them up. I stripped the wax stripped from the floors. For pizza and beer, friends helped me paint the apartment. Public Works passed the apartment; I was free to depart.

14

Icy Beaches

I marked my route in the atlas. Before leaving, a friend from New York helped me work out the best route and times to get around New York City to avoid as much traffic as possible when I left Momma's on the way to Rhode Island. My solo first road trip. Over the years, I would make many solo runs to see those I loved, but today I was nervous. When we traveled, Jim always drove. The drive to East St. Louis was just a few hours away. I'd stay there overnight before heading to Momma's.

While it wasn't a stick shift, driving the Fury was fun. With a 440 engine and four-barrel carburetor; it was fast and comfortable. I love a fast car. There was a CB in the car as well. Listening to the radio chatter, I could tell everyone thought I was an unmarked police officer. It took me two days to get to Momma's. Just as I'm nearly in her driveway, a motorcycle hit the rear passenger door. He wasn't seriously hurt, but Momma called an ambulance and the sheriff's department.

I didn't have any injuries, but the thought of admitting I had wrecked a car less than three months old had me physically shaking. Momma and I sat on the porch steps waiting for the sheriff to arrive. The motorcycle rider sat under a tree.

After collecting our statements, the deputy charged me with failure to yield right of way while making a left-hand turn. He totally ignored the yards of skid marks on the road made by the motorcycle and the fact that the door he hit was already in Momma's driveway when he hit it.

"Ma'am, since you're out of state and a military dependent without a permanent address, I'm to have going to take you in and hold you until we can get you before the magistrate. You'll have to post a thousand-dollar bond." He reached back for his handcuffs. "This is just procedure, ma'am."

I kept wringing my hands, struggling not to cry. "I have about twenty dollars in cash and my checkbook."

"Those out-of-state checks?"

"Yes, sir."

Momma had stayed on the porch but came walking up to us when she saw him reaching for the cuffs. "What's the matter, honey?"

As the deputy gets to the part about a thousand-dollar bond, Momma interrupts, "Let me make a phone call."

We all walk up to the porch. The deputy and I wait outside.

After just a few minutes, Momma steps to the door. "How much is her bail?"

"A thousand dollars, ma'am."

"If she pays the bail now, does she have to go to jail?"

"Ma'am, they won't take a check. Pardon me for asking, but how are you going to get a thousand dollars on Sunday night?"

"My sister owns the store down on the corner. She'll cash her check."

"Oh, I see. Well, since she has ties to the community and all, they'll probably just want five hundred. Get her car further up in the driveway and follow me. She can ride with you."

Abracadabra. Your aunt is a prominent businesswoman in the area. You skip ahead and pass go. No hand cuffs. No ride in the squad car. They cut the bail in half. Well, I got a couple of extra days with Momma and the kids as I dealt with the insurance company.

The delay put me behind on the trip. I wanted to be sure I was in Newport for Jim's graduation. So, I changed my route. Finishing the drive to Rhode Island was an eye opener and a test of nerves. First, there was the Francis Scott Key Bridge to get over. When I looked at the atlas, I realized the bridge was long, but taking it would cut hours off my trip. I neglected to realize its height, which let large ships pass through. Somehow, with white knuckles gripping the steering wheel, I made it over the bridge.

Next came New York. Nothing in life prepared me for the Cross Bronx Expressway. I had been talking with two truck drivers on the CB as I headed into New York City. Concerned that I was driving alone, they had me slip into the rocking chair and led me through New York. The sight of a car overturned in full flames on the wide median strip nearly undid me. No one was near the car, no police, no firefighters, and everyone kept driving.

All along the interstate stood the tall apartment buildings of the projects, which, even with a cursory glance, looked like hell on earth. I had seen similar things on the news but never in person. Over the next few years, I would take this route several times to see Momma in Virginia. It always made me question our humanity and wonder about ways to change a system which made these warrens possible.

In Connecticut, my truck driving companions veered off as I headed to a motel for the night. "Stay safe and get to that Navy man of yours. Maybe we'll catch you on the flip." I never knew their names, but I am forever grateful for their help.

Connecticut was a pleasant change of scenery. Pretty neighborhoods and forests. I made it to Jamestown, Rhode Island, and *damn, there's a bridge*. Another tall one to accommodate ships and sailboats. There's no way around it. Got to go over. White knuckles again.

I stayed at the Navy Lodge for about a week. Jim graduated. We attended a command cocktail party where I knew no one except Jim and just "milled about smartly," as my old captain had told me. We would stay in Newport on temporary duty for a time, so everything stayed in storage. Without household goods, we found a furnished apartment above a liquor store, a seasonal rental. It came equipped with everything and was just a short walk to the beach. Its rockiness seemed strange, the water was chilly, but there was sand and waves. I could see the ocean over the neighboring rooftops from my living room window.

I added to my cookbook collection. While there, I learned to cook Japanese and Chinese dishes in a wok. I cooked my second Thanksgiving meal there for a few friends who didn't go home for the holidays. This time, I made the gravy from scratch.

As if my last winter in Chicago wasn't bad enough, the weather thumbed its nose at me again. A blizzard closed the state. The Navy recalled Jim back to the base. Stuck in the apartment, I watched the scenes change outside my window. Waves lapped at a beach covered in ice and snow.

Snowmobiles were the only traffic, and there was a steady stream to the liquor store below. From my window, for the first time, I watched polar bear club adventurers as they plunged into the icy water. In the small marshy inlets where snow and ice covered the tall brown grasses left from summer, geese paddled to keep the water open. I passed the days watching the geese from my window or working on an embroidery project, hoping the weather would warm up so the geese could catch a break.

Eventually, the snow melted, and life returned to normal. The geese got to drier land. I found out I was pregnant. Excitedly, we called all the grandparents. Most were as excited as we were. I had hoped the news would be a way to find common ground with my dad, but he seemed less than pleased. "I'm too young to be a grandpa." He was young to have a daughter in her mid-twenties, none the less he disappointed me with this answer since it didn't sound like a joke.

Jim had orders. We were going to Virginia Beach.

I was excited to set up housekeeping and start entertaining as an officer's wife. Best of all, I'd be setting up a nursery. For once, I paid little attention to what was going on in the world around me.

15

Back Near a Warm Ocean

Although the ship was actually at Norfolk Naval Base, we looked for off base housing in Virginia Beach. We found a two-bedroom apartment with little trouble. Our household goods arrived. Jim had time to finish a rocking chair before he flew out to meet the ship.

The Officer's Wives Club was different here. There was a group for each ship. Much more informal than what I expected after my brief introduction in Great Lakes. We got together for lunch occasionally. I walked on the beach a lot during the off season.

I visited Momma several times. She and the boys had moved from Manassas to Shenandoah Farms. Terry now lived in Charlotte. After several years of working in her sister's store in Nokesville, Momma bought a small convenience store and gas station in the Farms. The first time, she met me in Nokesville, and I followed her to the store. I thought we would never get there. We visited around her time working in the store, and I helped with whatever project she had going on. It sat up the pattern for the rest of her life. Each of us helping the other when a need arose.

My pregnancy was uneventful except for morning sickness, which really lasted all day. When I talked to my doctor, he recommended eating small meals and snacking on saltines throughout the day. They no longer prescribed a medication for this. In the 1950s and 1960s, there was a widely used medication for morning sickness. Tragically, it led to terrible birth defects. These children came to be known as thalidomide babies. I gladly suffered with saltines and ginger ale.

Drugs during pregnancy became an abomination to me. In the seventies, deliveries without routine drugs and having the father in the delivery room were a new practice. I had I already learned I didn't process drugs well. Besides, the Tylenol scare was in full swing. Although they were coming into vogue, I didn't think home births were safe. What if there was an emergency?

I read Dr. Lamaze's books about "natural childbirth" which favored fewer drugs during the delivery. It also encouraged fathers to be present as a coach and so they could bond with the baby sooner. I had found my answer. To have this type of delivery in a naval hospital, both parents had to go to classes and present a certificate to the hospital.

Momma fully embraced her role as a grandmother, even though she was in her late thirties when her first grandchild was born. She made the trip from Front Royal to Virginia Beach and helped me set up the nursery. We found Winnie the Pooh curtains for the nursery and a bassinet. At a fabric store, we purchased yards of white eyelet and yellow ribbon to make a skirt for the bassinet.

Back at the apartment, Momma talked me through the steps for making a simple lining for the bassinet and attaching the eyelet. We hung the Winnie the Pooh curtains together. I would put the lining and skirt together after she left.

During a break, she told me. "I want the children to call me 'Grandmother'. Then there's no confusion and we always know who they're talking about."

"Well, okay Momma. It might be hard at first. That's a big word for little kids." I smiled at her, knowing she always wanted to be known for who she was.

"Of course, but they'll get the hang of it. Oh, let me get that bag from the car. And how about making some coffee?"

Momma came back inside as I set our coffee mugs on the dinette table. "I was by the consignment store the other day and I got these outfits. I bought the bigger size because everyone will buy those cute little newborn things. Baby will outgrow those in no time."

By now she's nothing like the quiet woman I grew up with. Multiple rings with gemstones flashed on her fingers. She would dress to the nines and go to local dances. Occasionally, her sisters would try to get her to "tone it down". "If Dolly Parton can wear all her makeup and those wigs, I can do what I want," was her reply.

I took a class to learn how to crochet and made the three potholders. Try as I might, I couldn't translate this knowledge into a sweater. It came out looking like a trapezoid rather than a square. My sewing and embroidery skills were fine, so I busied myself making outfits and embroidering my first quilt for the basinet.

I read everything I could find about the care and feeding of infants to include contamination problems with commercial baby food. When the baby was ready, I had a food grinder so I could make healthy food. I wanted everything to be as natural as possible.

In those days, military couples relied on mail to keep in touch. No email. No face time or zoom. Upon the advice from another wife, I numbered my letters as mail delivery to ships was erratic and letters often arrived out of order. Occasionally, there were ham radio calls patched into the phone system. You had to remember to say "over" at the end of your sentence, so the other person knew when to key their mike and talk. Also, the entire communications department and any-one with a ham radio heard everything you said, so there were never any intense or private conversations.

I never got used to waiting on the pier for Jim to get off the ship. You had to get there early to find a parking spot close to the pier. There was no place to sit as we waited for the sailors to moor the ship to the dock and lower the gangplank. The entire process was tedious. Then you have to walk up the gangplank. Empty supply ships sit high in the water. Often once the gangplank was down, a sailor would escort me to the wardroom to wait for Jim to wrap up his day. At least I wasn't still standing on the pier.

Sometimes the swirl of emotions---not just your own but those of other women and children waiting was a palpable, living thing wrapping everyone in its tentacles. Anticipation so thick it clogged the air, wrapped around your throat and threatened to cut off your breath. Will I recognize him? Does he have a still have his mustache? Will he recognize me now that I'm eight months pregnant? For some resignation---here we are again.

The return from deployments can be like a honeymoon. Even with the positives, it's a disruption of the wife's routine which kept things together during the deployment. If he has any rank and especially as an officer, he's used to people doing what he says. Reintegrating the navy man back into his family can be a complicated dance even in peacetime.

In the seventies, many doctors felt "the longer the baby stays in the womb, the better". My due date came, and time went on by. Jim's parents called daily to see if I was in labor and if not, why not? *How do I know? This is my first baby.* I walked. I cried. I kept yet another obstetrics appointment.

After a few bouts of false labor, I made it to the labor room. I had only been in labor a short time when Jimmy started showing signs of distress. His heart rate was up, and the doctor thought he wasn't getting enough oxygen. I received medication to speed up my labor. There was very little build up, just hard contractions.

At last, the final push. I held him for just a few moments. Then the nurses whisked him off to the Neonatal Intensive Care Unit (NICU) because he was a blue baby. Other nurses trundled me off to my room downstairs. I was expecting him to arrive at my bedside in the morning. Even though I had signed up for rooming in, hospital policy had all babies returned to the nursery at night.

After breakfast, I became more anxious. "Where's my baby?" I asked the nurse. "I'm supposed to be rooming in."

"Didn't anyone tell you? He's in the NICU. I'm sorry. Let me get the pediatrician for you."

I waited, tears welled up and rolled down my cheeks. Even though I had a normal ultrasound a few months ago, I imagined many terrible things. *Will Jimmy be okay? What did I eat? What did I do?* Jim was at work. I paced around the room from bed to chair and back. From the window, I couldn't see the old trees on the hospital grounds, just the side of another building. Nothing to help calm me.

"Mrs. Denam, I'm Dr. Walters. I'm taking care of your baby while you're in the hospital. Let me explain. Then I'll get someone to take you up to the NICU once I get the spinal tap."

Jimmy was hypoxic because his cord had wrapped around his neck. The doctors placed him under an oxygen hood on his back to ensure he took in the oxygen. He vomited, aspirated, and had a seizure. Now they were trying to determine if he had a seizure disorder. He was being given medication to control seizures, which made him very sleepy. Dr. Walters thought hypoxia following aspiration caused Jimmy's seizure.

There was a parent's room connected to the NICU. The walls were glass so the nurses could observe in case of an emergency. After scrubbing and gowning up, I entered the nursery. At nine pounds six ounces and 21 inches long, Jimmy barely fit in the layette. After a couple of days, they brought Jimmy in his layette out into the parent's room, so I'd have all his supplies for my visits. I'd spend most of the day with him.

Although I was planning to breastfeed, the nurses gave him formula during the night. With a nurse's help, I gave him his first feeding from the breast. Then I rocked him, singing "Summertime" until the nurses told me the doctors were rounding on the maternity ward.

Over the next two weeks, a pattern developed. I had breakfast on the ward and then up to the NICU to feed, play with Jimmy, and pump milk for the nighttime feedings while Jimmy slept. Downstairs for obstetric rounds, back upstairs for pediatric rounds, time with Jimmy, lunch downstairs and then back upstairs. The electric pump on the NICU was just under three feet tall and about eighteen inches wide. You pumped just one breast at a time. Modern breast pumps are so much nicer, more efficient.

Giving birth was such a transcendent experience for me, but also terrifying. Now I'm responsible for another human. My persistent questioning of myself, the responsibility and having an infant in a NICU was almost crushing. *Did I eat the wrong thing? What about me made the umbilical cord wrap around his neck? Can I take care of him at home so he develops as he should?* It was also a humbling experience. *If I'm terrified, how must the mothers of the little preemies feel? At least I know Jimmy will come home soon. To have to wait for months would be dreadful.*

Dr. Walters was an amazing pediatrician. He encouraged me to provide much of Jimmy's care in the hospital. He and the nurses gave me a lot of positive feedback while shielding me from things like Jimmy's spinal tap. I saw a spinal tap later when the staff forgot to pull the screen. The doctor holds the baby up by one foot, dangles him over the layette—to keep the spine straight. Even before the puncture, the baby was screaming.

Jim came by in the evening after work. We'd have dinner in the cafeteria. Then we'd visit with Jimmy before he headed back to Virginia Beach.

During the night, I would pump every two hours and send it to the NICU. When Jimmy was two weeks old, I had to go home without him. They needed my bed for an expected influx of maternity patients. I was forever thankful I could stay so long since I needed absolutely no nursing or medical care.

For the first few days after I left the hospital, Jim took me to the hospital on his way to the ship. In the evening, he spent time with Jimmy and then took me home. When the ship left port for exercises, I cried. I wasn't supposed to drive yet. *If I can't get to the hospital, how would Jimmy know I loved him and hadn't just left him?* I continued pumping at home with a less efficient hand-held bulb syringe pump and learned to freeze it in ice cube trays. I was determined to have a supply when he came home. The hospital used what I pumped when I was there.

Momma came to drive me back and forth to the hospital in Portsmouth so I could see him daily. We would spend all day caring for him before returning home to sleep and go back the next day. By this time, Dr. Walters felt sure Jimmy didn't have a seizure disorder. Weaning him off the phenobarbital would be a slow process. I would finish that at home. Momma and I brought him home when he was nearly three weeks old. After a couple of days, Momma returned to Front Royal.

Now Jimmy and I are on our own. The phenobarbital was so sedating; I had to wake Jimmy up for each feeding and encourage him to stay awake. Change his diaper, range of motion, feeding, burping. Keep him awake, encourage him to track things within his field of vision.

Eventually, it all became routine. At each visit, Dr. Walters would make sure Jimmy was hitting his development milestones and review the next stage of development. We tailored Jimmy's exercise routine to help him meet the next developmental milestones. Things like when to offer Cheerios to develop a pincer grasp or when to introduce blocks. Jimmy was off phenobarbital by his first birthday, and he was pulling up as he got ready to walk.

Jim wasn't home for long periods of time. He had transferred to another ship and was frequently out for fleet exercises. I began understanding how to run a home. Getting all the bills paid. Keeping it clean. Running all the errands. All this while making Jimmy's baby food from fresh vegetables, juggling his appointments, and exercise routines. Before this, I had followed Jim's lead for most things.

I found a good babysitter and started classes at Tidewater Community College. I was trying to find a career compatible with Jim's future career moves. Jim was positive about me going to school. Later, it would be the timing of my return to the workforce would cause difficulty. Thinking of the civilians working at the dental center in Great Lakes, I started out on a secretarial track, shorthand, and such. As a veteran, I would have some advantages in the civil service system. The coursework was boring. Before even completing my first quarter and on the advice of a counselor, I shifted to business administration with a focus on accounting.

I had classes three days a week. All early morning, so I'd have the afternoon with Jimmy. With Jimmy in a sling, I walked on the beach. I read books to him all the time. When he napped in the afternoon, I studied. The apartment was small, so there wasn't a problem keeping up with housework.

It was good to be with other adults. Ones that had nothing to do with my husband's career. To laugh and joke without thinking of any judgement. As always, I was pretty focused on schoolwork. I breezed through the general studies portion of the curriculum, which was not as challenging as my Myers Park course work had been. I attended school year-round since I wanted to complete the associate degree before Jim came up for transfer.

Although his orders were uncertain, we moved to a four-bedroom townhouse so our second child would have their own room. All the bedrooms and a full bathroom upstairs and a powder room downstairs. I remember thinking having two bathrooms meant you were moving up in the world. No Navy move this time. It was a matter of packing up and renting a U-Haul truck. At this stage of the game, it was simple since we had gained little in the way of household goods.

During my second year at Tidewater Community College (TCC), I became pregnant. Not so much morning sickness this time. However, I worried about having problems like those I had with Jimmy and having enough love for another baby. I talked to Momma on the phone several times a week. Usually in the evening, after long distance telephone rates were lower.

"Momma, how do you know you can love all your children? I love Jimmy so much. How can I love another baby as much as I love Jimmy?"

Thank goodness she didn't laugh. "A mother's heart just grows with all her babies. Each time, you find your heart grows. None of them will be the same. As they grow, you see the things that make each one special to you. Things that take nothing away from the others." Even with her reassurance, these thoughts troubled me throughout my pregnancy.

David was also born at Portsmouth Naval Hospital—but the new one. Here all the rooms were birthing rooms. David arrived safely nine pounds, four ounces and 23 inches long. The first time I held him in my arms, I knew Momma was right. Your heart just grows and envelopes your tiny new human. No need for the NICU, just rooming in for three days and home. Jim was home for a week and then out to exercises again. Momma and Martin visited for a short time.

When David was about nine months old, I returned to TCC to finish my Associates. Taking biology made me dream of the medical and nursing field, but I held to the set course set and finished on the Dean's List. At least all the courses would be transferable to a four-year university whenever I could go back for my bachelors.

The next few months found me feeling isolated. School was over for now. The boys and I spent time at the pool in the complex. I didn't want them to be afraid of the water like I was. I didn't socialize with the officer's wives too much. You always had to be so careful of what you said and how you did things. Once again, I didn't fit in.

The children and I often visited Momma in Front Royal when the ship wasn't in port. I'd help behind the register while she played with the boys. We would drive into Manassas and hit the thrift stores. After the store closed and the boys were sleeping, we'd work on her latest project to transform the store and have a few drinks. Usually, I'd stay for a weekend.

That winter, Jim got orders for training in Rhode Island. After the Navy shipped our household goods, we took a trip to Louisiana to see his parents. We traveled in two cars. We had Christmas there before going up to Virginia to see Momma.

We had a few days with Momma before heading to Newport. As we were loading up to leave, sleet started falling. Jim felt the sleet would end soon, and we headed out as planned. Before we got out of Front Royal, my left windshield wiper broke. Nothing was open. And Jim had to report on time. So, he tied a cord to the windshield wiper and the steering wheel so I could operate the windshield wiper manually by pulling the string. It was a long trip, but we made it in the day allotted even with stops for the boys.

16

Ocean Swales

This time, we had base housing from the beginning. The officer's section, at least, looked much like any suburban community---curving streets with lots of trees near the houses. The houses were mostly duplexes with some single-family homes for more senior officers. We had a three-bedroom duplex with a living room, dining room, kitchen, and powder room downstairs. Hardwood floors ran throughout the unit. There was a carport and an outside storage room. A playground was just a short walk up a hill in the common area. The local dairy even made deliveries in the neighborhood.

Momma gave us a cherry wood dining room table and chairs. The table had a double pedestal base with folding sides and three additional leaves. Fully extended, it would seat twelve. After rubbing it down with some Old English polish, it looked especially beautiful. I recovered the chair seats once Jim had refinished them.

At first, I was excited to be in housing; I hoped to find the sense of community I had known in Great Lakes. We set up a barter system for babysitting. It was nice if you wanted to leave Newport for shopping. Sometimes I used it. Mostly, I took the boys with me whenever I shopped. I met Sue; she and her husband were in California before. She taught me how to make my own patterns and sew stretchy knits like T-shirts and shorts. They avoided most functions. They were really into ecology and saving the planet. Our children played together well.

"Sue, are you going to the afternoon tea next Wednesday?" I asked as we were sewing together at my dining room table. The children played nearby.

"No, I don't think so. I'm not really into that stuff. I can watch the boys if you want to go."

"Maybe I will. I'm just trying to get used to this officer business. Everything seems a lot different from our being enlisted. Jim thinks I need to get involved with the wives' club."

The day of the tea found me staring at my closet, trying to figure out what to wear. Obviously, I couldn't wear jeans. Wearing a dress seemed too formal. Finally, I settled on a navy Eva Picone pantsuit with low pumps that I had picked up at the Exchange. After dropping the boys off, I arrived at Shelby's a few minutes early.

"Oh, hi Sherry. I'm so glad you could make it. Come in." Shelby said, opening the door and taking my coat. "Grab yourself something to eat and drink. Everything is in the dining room."

Several women already sat in the living room. Everything was gorgeous. The layout of her unit was like mine, but her furniture looked as if they had transported it straight from an Ethan Allen showroom. They had covered the ubiquitous black asphalt tile with nearly wall to wall rugs. Shelby had arranged a silver tea service, china cups and saucers on the buffet. The china was ornate. Yellow and white flowers filled a pale gray border with gold trim. Light appetizers, set out in crystal and silver dishes, surrounded a fresh floral arrangement on the dining room table. She had set everything up precisely as described in the etiquette books I'd read. It was beautiful.

When I complimented Shelby on her china pattern, she replied offhandedly, "Oh, that was my grandmother's Lenox set. She gave it to me when John and I married." Her tone implied that grandmother had several sets of china.

Briefly, we talked about our husband's previous duty stations. One woman asked when Jim graduated. When I mentioned OSC, she remarked, "Ah, that's why I didn't recognize your name. Mike went to Annapolis" and turned to speak to someone else.

The talk turned to shopping in Providence for the latest styles "Because you can't find anything in the Exchange". Even then, I didn't have an interest in shopping as an activity. You shopped because you needed something, not because there was nothing else to do.

At one point, I tried to talk about returning to school, but most of them had already graduated from college. No one seemed interested in returning to work and looked skeptically at me as I mentioned working when the boys were older.

"Oh, no. There are so many things to do with the club, house, and children. We support the men and keep everything going," Shelby said. "Some people sell Tupperware and Mary Kay. But you shouldn't. It's better just to focus on helping your husband advance his career. It is hard sometimes being far away from your family, but you get used to it after a while. Just don't go around moping. That's not going to help anyone."

School was mentally intense for the men. As usual, placement in the class was a major factor in obtaining your desired duty station. Where the next duty station would be was becoming an issue. Jim wanted to go to the west coast to be further away from the east coast bureaucracy. I wanted to go back to Virginia. I had already experienced the loneliness of waiting for the ship to return to port and didn't want to do that again with phone calls as my only link to family. Besides, I didn't like San Diego the first time around. I missed the seasons and a gentler flow to life.

I spent my days putting the house together, doing embroidery projects and playing with the boys---gathering seashells as we walked along the beaches or at the playground. There was the occasional Tupperware or Mary Kay party to break things up. I began making purchases for things considered a "must have" for entertaining in a naval officer's world. I purchased my Mikasa china there because I liked the shape of the cup. With black and platinum bands on white, its understated design was not too ornate. It fit in nicely with my eclectic tastes.

Also, through the Navy Exchange, I bought my linen tablecloth and napkins. Jim's parents given us had a suitable set of stainless flatware when he graduated from Officer Candidate School. Momma gave us a sterling silver tea service she had purchased with S&H green stamps. She began scouring the thrift stores for silver serving dishes with glass inserts to use on a buffet.

We had fellow students and their families over. Nothing formal. We grilled something or steamed seafood. Jim usually manned the grill, but I learned to grill a pretty good London broil. After we ate, the wives would gather with the children while the men played games. The games usually involved a military strategy. Often the games were still going strong after the wives and children left and I had put the boys to bed.

I began having cluster headaches. They were nearly disabling. Probably would have been if it weren't for the boys. For them, I got up every day. Fixed the meals, cleaned the house, took them outside, read and built towers with Legos. But when they napped, I napped, always hoping that I could sleep longer. I gained weight.

Eventually, I made an appointment at the dispensary to get something for my headaches. After running a few tests and finding nothing organically amiss, the doctor talked to me about what was happening in my life. And depression.

"I see nothing in your test results that would cause your headaches. So, what's going on at home? Your husband is here for school? Does he have orders yet?"

"Yes, we've got another three months here. We have two boys, four and two. They keep me pretty busy. No orders. We're just talking about places he's considering."

"What do you think about the choices?"

"I'd like to stay on the east coast because I have family in Virginia, and he wants to move to the west coast. I don't feel like I have much choice in the matter."

He gave me information about dietary changes that might decrease my headaches. "Think you need to talk seriously with your husband about your next duty station. You'll be a better support if you are happy with the choices, and you'll feel better, too. Once your mood improves, you may find that you have fewer headaches."

"So, what about my weight?"

"Right now, focus on the headaches and working out the duty station situation. Once you and your husband decide on the next duty station, start logging what you eat and then count the calories. When you have your intake logged, you can figure what to cut out without harming your nutrition." This was an unusual exchange for a visit with a military doctor. He was definitely ahead of his time.

Jim and I eventually came to an agreement about staying on the east coast. I found that caffeine restriction wasn't the answer to my headaches. My body was so used to caffeine that being without it made the headaches more severe. Once I resumed my normal caffeine intake and the decision about duty stations resolved, I no longer had headaches. At last, school was over. We received orders back to Virginia Beach.

Raised by a strong woman and being invested in the women's movement gave me a sense that I needed to develop myself besides being a mother and wife. My plan was to stay home until the boys were well into elementary school and then return to work. However, the expectation was that I would remain home, raise the children, and present the picture of a perfect life to all the world, even if things weren't perfect. It was almost funny to find the British stiff upper lip alive and well in the US Navy. Except it wasn't. I blithely carried on with life, still not understanding the connection between physical and mental health.

17

Choppy Seas

Before leaving Newport, we contacted a real estate agent who located a few rental homes in Virginia Beach for us to check out. Luckily, we found a house next door to a couple Jim met in OCS. It would be nice to have a neighbor we knew.

Open floor plans weren't a thing then, but this was close. You entered straight into a combined living room and dining room. The wall separating the large eat-in kitchen ended about two feet from the ceiling. Sliding doors in the kitchen led to the backyard. The master was on the ground floor with a large walk-in closet. Jack and jill doors gave access to the downstairs full bath from the master bedroom. A small downstairs room served as the den and playroom for the boys. Upstairs, there were three bedrooms and another full bathroom. Wall to wall carpeting was everywhere except the kitchen and bathrooms. There was an attached garage. More house than I had ever dealt with.

Wall units we had originally purchased as bookshelves served as a display area for the room. One section had a drop-down door that served as a bar. The closed areas on the bottom stored china and serving pieces. Mom found a nice couch and chair. A friend brought them down from Front Royal. I found an inexpensive chair, brass and glass coffee table and end tables to round out the living room area. I made a casual tablecloth for the dining room table from a bedsheet. Jim's mother had given us an embroidered tablecloth, but I saved it for special family occasions.

By the time we had the furniture arranged, Jim was back at sea. Again, I was spending time at the beach with the boys or with the occasional wives' club function. Like most wives, I watched CNN anytime the boys weren't in the room. I kept logging my food intake but wasn't showing results as quickly as I liked. I was just marking the days trying to figure out where life was going. The seas were choppy, but I was holding on.

Momma and Aunt Vivian came down for a few days. Aunt Vivian was so excited to visit the Edgar Casey Center. The mystical and alternative medicines always fascinated her. After talking with Momma, I found a good preschool and started back to school.

I enrolled in Old Dominion University and minored in computer science along with my major in business administration. Classroom discussions and general conversation with adults who spoke freely invigorated me. The boys and I had a good routine. Three days a week they were in preschool, and I picked them up after class. Since they had an eight o'clock bedtime, it was easy to study once the boys were asleep. My weight loss efforts were showing results.

During hurricane David, the Navy sent all ships out to sea to weather the storm. The initial plan was for the boys and me to stay in Virginia Beach. As the hurricane drew closer, I rethought this plan. The Hampton Roads tunnel connected Norfolk and Virginia Beach to Hampton Roads and Newport News. Traffic delays were common during normal times. Concerned about being in a potential disaster area with two small children, I went to Momma's without waiting for an official evacuation order. While I was there, Momma introduced me to depression glass. She had several bought pieces at estate sales. She kept a few and sold the others.

While we were there, Momma cooked a big dinner. She still cooked in the old Southern tradition: fried chicken, veggies swimming in bacon grease, pies, and cakes. It always amazed me by how she could stretch food and make gravy from anything. When I was younger, she would heat the cast-iron skillet, add a couple of sliced up hot dogs with some fatback grease and make a gravy. Much like chipped beef or sausage gravy. She'd serve it over grits. If there were extra grits, she spread them in a loaf pan and put them in the refrigerator. Later she would slice the grits and in fry them in fatback grease. We ate it with margarine and syrup. "Just like pancakes" she'd say. She taught me how to cook as I grew up, but like many young women, I didn't have the confidence to carry out her some of her recipes like cornbread stuffing or scratch made chocolate pie.

Too soon, the boys and I had to return to Virginia Beach. I wasn't really excited about the idea. More of the sameness of every day. More uncertainty about the future. I made plans to come back for Thanksgiving. The ships returned to port.

In no time at all, Jim was on deployment again. I started falling asleep with the television tuned to CNN. Things were warming up in the Middle East again and the ship was cruising in the Mediterranean. Rumors flew around like starlings to a bird feeder. You'd think you figured out the situation. Then a new rumor swooped in, turning things upside down. Then, with raucous calls, another bird took its place. A vicious circle. Senior officer's wives tried to reassure us that everything would be okay. In the end, they were right, but anxiety and stress levels were high. We all watched CNN thinking we could garner some clue at about our loved ones.

The boys and I went to Momma's for Thanksgiving. It was good to see my brothers and sister. This year I was determined to learn how to make Momma's cornbread stuffing.

"That cornbread should be ready. Take it out, cut it up and turn the slices on their side so they can cool some."

Together, we chopped up the celery and onion. "Be sure to chop them up small."

"Like this Momma?"

"Yes, that's it. Okay, let's crumble up that cornbread, add the turkey stock and get things mixed up. Just dig in with your hands."

"Alright" At first, I tried mixing it with a large spoon, but Momma was right. You needed to dig in with both hands.

I mixed everything up except the sage. "How much sage do you use, Momma?"

"Shake some in and taste it. If it doesn't taste right, keep adding sage until it does. Some people like to put their dressing in the turkey. I don't because bacteria from the turkey might not get killed in the stuffing, and we'd all get food poisoning."

Too soon, we were back in Virginia Beach and still sleeping with the TV on, I began incorporating news broadcasts into my dreams. In a vivid dream, I saw the ship blown up on television. I woke up in a cold sweat, my heart pounding as I sobbed hysterically at two in the morning. I turned off the television. It was some time before I could calm down and go back to sleep.

By the time Jim returned from deployment, he didn't recognize me on the pier. I was back down to my weight when I entered the Navy. I was proud and pleased with myself. With a few hiccups, we established a new routine as I continued with classes, and he came home most nights. The exception being when he had duty and remained onboard ship. On those nights, the boys and I often had dinner in the wardroom. Sometimes another family would be there.

Eating in the wardroom was an experience. One large table dominated the wardroom and off to the side there was a lounge area with couches and smaller tables for playing cards. At mealtimes, a tablecloth covered the larger table. Everyone had cloth napkins rolled into napkin rings. The officers had their initials engraved in theirs as they used their napkins for a full day. The food was pretty good. Mess cooks served us as we sat at the table. After coffee, there was often a movie.

The honeymoon period didn't last so long this time. He became frustrated with the politics within the Navy, and I had learned to be more assertive. We either didn't talk or we argued.

Despite this, Christmas that year was more like what I felt Christmas should be. Although we had small trees once Jimmy was born, Jim wasn't as into Christmas decorating as I was. This year, we had a large tree in the living room and stockings hanging over the fireplace. The boys and I made cookies.

The boys' shouts of glee on Christmas Day made everything worthwhile. "I got everything I wanted," they called out as they opened their presents. I resolved then never again to be so complete in checking off Santa's list. I didn't have any plans, but I was sure the time would come when Santa wouldn't be able to deliver everything on their lists.

By spring, things in our relationship came to a head. An old friend from our days in Great Lakes suggested counseling. In the seventies, divorce and counseling for any problem carried an enormous stigma. This was especially true in the military. Also, for counseling to work, both parties must be amenable. I kept appointments for a few of the counseling sessions. Not in good faith, I must admit. In ten years, I had given all I had and wanted the counselor to help me make Jim see it.

Determined that what happened in the marriage would stay between Jim and me; I tried to stay in Virginia Beach so that it would be easier for the boys to see Jim. Unlike me, Jimmy and David could know and make their own decisions about their dad as they grew up. Everything had been in Jim's name, so he could take advantage of Illinois residency at tax time. I had no real credit history. I had not worked since I was in the Navy.

The boys and I moved to a townhouse near friends of mine. The owner wanted to sell it but was happy to give me a short-term lease as I sorted things out. Momma came down to help me get settled. Eventually, we moved into a house shared with another friend.

I tried to find a job doing anything. McDonald's turned me down as being overqualified. I briefly worked at a staffing agency. There, the manager gave her friends the accounts that paid well. I finally found a job as a bill collector for a jewelry store and became fairly good at skip tracing. Skip tracing involves figuring out how to reach a customer who was no longer paying their bill and getting them to restart payments. Curious work considering we didn't have the internet. We searched through old records and making notes of what we found. I also worked wrapping gifts in a high-end department store on weekends when the boys were with Jim.

My Fury had developed serious engine problems, so I sold it for scrap. I purchased a ten-year-old Ford Galaxy so I could get back and forth to work. Wouldn't you know, the starter stopped working when I was short of cash. A friend took me to the library where I looked in a Chilton's and found the steps for changing a starter. Thankfully, Jim stored his tools in my garage. It took me all morning, cussing, crying, and crawling around under the car to get the job done. But I did it.

Jimmy was in first grade. I traded babysitting with a neighbor who worked opposite hours from me. Each morning, I dropped David at her house and Jimmy off at school. She picked Jimmy up from school and watched both boys until I got off work. It worked out well until she moved to a day shift. For a couple of weeks, David played in the back room of the jewelry store while I made calls. I had to work fewer hours so that I could pick Jimmy up after school.

Virginia Beach was an expensive place to live. I didn't make enough to support the boys and myself, even with Jim's child support. I didn't receive alimony, as we were filing under Virginia's "no fault" laws. Jim was getting ready for shore duty, but not sure where he'd be stationed. He agreed to make the separation legal under Virginia law and to my moving to Front Royal with Jimmy and David. This would let me help Momma in the store, since her respiratory illness was getting worse. I would have childcare, family support, a regular paycheck, and a ho

18

Snakes and Floods

Momma's store was about thirty minutes outside Front Royal at the intersection of two state roads. The store stocked a fair selection of grocery items and the usual convenience store items. It had a snack bar serving breakfast and sandwiches. After work, people would stop in for something to eat, drink a few beers and shoot pool.

Most people in the community worked in construction, although a few people had office jobs in Manassas and DC. Homes in the bedroom communities of Manassas and Warrenton had become more expensive. There were a lot of weekend homes and since there was a state park nearby, the weekends were busy. As in many small communities, most people were related one way or the other and had lived there for a few generations.

Momma opened the store at six in the morning so people could get gas and coffee on their way to work. During hunting season, we would open at five. Since Momma opened, I could get the boys on the school bus and get a few things done in the apartment. I would overlap Momma's shift to help stock and closed the store around ten.

The boys often did their homework and ate dinner upstairs while things were quiet. As people began drifting to the pool table, Jimmy and David would go downstairs with Momma. The store's layout made working alone difficult. You couldn't see the snack bar area from the cash register. Working the evenings involved going back and forth from the store to the snack bar to serve beer and be sure no one was overtly gambling while playing pool. It could get hectic.

When the boys and I first moved to Front Royal, we shared Momma and Martin's two-bedroom apartment below the store. All my things were in a storage shed. Shortly afterward, we began creating an apartment for Momma and Martin in what were originally two large garage bays. We hired out the plumbing, electricity, and framing. Momma and I helped with things like paneling and flooring.

Once she and Martin were in their own apartment, I started work in the boys' room. Wallpaper was expensive, I used adhesive shelf liner to cover the walls. Its grid pattern of red, yellow, and blue on a white background really brightened up the room. I purchased bunk beds and a chest of drawers from this End Up. I also hired a babysitter for the evenings I worked. Momma didn't mind watching the boys, but I wanted her to rest. They were my responsibility.

Water damage ruined my stored sofa, so I purchased a new gray one from Schwell's on a payment plan. I repainted the living room a medium gray. A friend recovered a chair from a thrift store with fabric I found on sale at JOANN fabrics. I hung rose-colored sheers in the living room.

After paying bills, I would go to a small bookstore in Front Royal. I'd buy a book for myself and one for each of the boys. I bought my first copy of Writer's Market there. I bought a used Selectric typewriter and began submitting stories to various women's magazines. So many rejections. No publication.

It wasn't all work. The boys and I went to the playground in town. Every so often, we'd stop at McDonald's afterwards. People were always going to the river to fish. The boys were curious about fishing, but after Wayne's death, I couldn't face watching them near the river. I took them up to the trout farm where we fished with simple rod and reels.

I also wanted them to be well rounded and self-sufficient. They were already learning to help with household chores, but I tried to be sensitive to the fact that there weren't many active male role models in their life, so I included "manly" activities in their lives. Jim was with them every other weekend and, in the summer, but they spent their time watching movies or playing video games. Besides, fishing made me remember fun times with my grandpa.

Momma was having more trouble with her asthma. After a couple of rounds of antibiotics, she was in the hospital with pneumonia. I was constantly on the go from Winchester, Front Royal, and the store. Momma loathed wearing hospital gowns "I feel so exposed" so I bought her pretty jewel tone-colored pajamas from Peebles.

My mind on Momma, I got up one morning, pulled on some clothes, started out of my bedroom door, and jumped back on the bed. Just outside the door, heading into my room, was a copperhead snake. Shivers convulsed my body. My heart racing, I froze. *Oh, the boys are in their room. How am I going to get to them?* I bunched up my comforter, threw it over the snake, and launched myself into the hall. Sprinting down the hall, I shook the boys awake.

"Come on, guys. Get your clothes on. We've got to go outside. There's a snake in the apartment."

My heart still pounding, I get the boys upstairs to the store.

"Liz, a copperhead got into the apartment. Do you know how to get rid of it?"

"I've heard they'll go away from mothballs. I don't know if it works, though."

Hurrying over to a shelf in the store, I grab the six boxes of mothballs we have on the shelf. "Hey, put these on my tab."

"Yeah, I got it. I'll fix the boys something to eat in the snack bar and keep them upstairs."

"Thanks."

I run back downstairs, grab a hoe and shovel as I get to the apartment door. My belly is churning. Feeling a little dizzy, I realize I'm holding my breath. *Breathe.* I force myself to go into the apartment. Using the hoe, I lift the comforter from the floor. No snake.

One room at a time, I flip on the lights and sprinkle moth balls. I try to leave an exit path to the door for the snake. No snake. I can't see under some of the furniture. Breathless, I climb on my desk and pull my feet under me. I take a small trash can up with me. Between the moth balls and thinking about the snake, my stomach is turning like a cement mixer.

Still no snake in sight.

Sitting cross-legged on the desk, I call the Agriculture Extension office and discuss my problem. "No, ma'am, we don't do snake removals." They offer no advice other than to call a company that removed animals from your home. *I don't have the money for that.* I went back to watching the floor.

The snake finally began moving sluggishly into the office area. Shaking so hard I can barely hold on to the hoe, I try to herd the snake towards the open door while still sitting on the desk. I nearly fall to the floor when the phone rings.

"Hear you got a snake?" From his tone, I can tell Ben is grinning from ear to ear.

"Yeah, I can see it now" I gave Ben a rundown of events. "Oh, damn, he's going back towards my bedroom."

"Let me call someone. I got a buddy crazy enough to hunt out that snake. We'll get it out Sis."

About a half an hour later, Ben and Joe knocked on the door.

"Come on in. I don't know where the snake is now. It went off down the hall."

"Sis, just hang out with the boys upstairs. I'll come get you when we're done."

"Okay, thanks Ben." I force myself to get off the desk and run out the door.

After a bit, Ben calls upstairs. "Look out the back window."

Looking out the window, I see Joe standing in the middle of the yard, holding two three-foot snakes just below their heads. Later, Ben and I poked around the apartment for a good while, trying to figure out how the snakes got in. No luck.

Later, I found out that Angie, my babysitter, had opened the doors to the apartment the night before because she didn't want to turn on the AC. Ben put up screen doors for me soon after.

I didn't enjoy working evenings when the pool table was busy. I never developed Momma's knack for harmless flirtation and chatter. As the new girl in town, I heard every pickup line in the book. Which wouldn't have been so bad, but it never stopped, and they were never clever. "Wanna grab a six-pack and go down by the river?" was typical or "You'd be really pretty if you would smile more". My sarcastic response "Only idiots smile all the time" did not win me friends. I was not interested in dating. I just wanted to raise my two sons.

If I just had to serve beer, it wouldn't have been so bad. But I had to watch everyone to be sure they weren't taking their beer out to the porch, having a little toke, or lifting a "free" six pack from the store on their way out. Then there were the fights. Most of the time, other patrons would put a stop to things.

One Saturday night, Gene was drinking pretty heavily and hitting on every woman in sight. He had obviously been drinking before he got there. One woman's boyfriend got pretty upset, and they started tussling, not really fighting.

"Gene, Ralph, knock it off you two. Take it outside." I yell from behind the counter as I got a beer for another customer.

Gene turns his attention to me. Crossing the room, he yells, "No stuck-up bitch is going to tell me what to do."

We kept a Berretta and a pool stick behind the counter. I flipped the pool stick handle away from me and hit the counter hard. The loud crack silenced the room.

"Get out now before I call the sheriff. Don't think you want them searching your car."

He left, yelling obscenities, and throwing gravel against the building as he sped out of the parking lot.

It was a royal pain but the pool table introduced me to Keith, my future second husband. He would shoot pool and have a few beers on his way home from work. Keith and his brother owned a house close to the river. He asked me out a few times, to dinner and a movie. I turned him down. He stopped asking. Keith still came into the store, always with a joke.

There was serious flooding that spring, and several people lost their homes that were close to the river. While we were not in danger from the water, flooding and fallen trees blocked the road to town. We worried about losing grocery store stock when we lost power for a short time. Fortunately, it wasn't out for long, as I could not find dry ice within fifty miles of the store.

As the water receded, we began having trouble with our well's pump. Momma was the queen of the barter system. Often getting work done for a bit of cash and a case or two of beer. Keith helped a few times by pulling the pump. Then we didn't see him or Todd for several weeks. Word had it that flooding destroyed their house by the river.

Momma and I added a dinner menu in the snack-bar. Simple home style meals. Eat in or take out. Besides being another draw during the slower weekdays, it helped us balance the amount of food served with the amount of beer sold for on premise consumption. Otherwise, we ran into trouble with ABC regulations.

Keith returned from Pennsylvania. He often ate dinner at the snack bar before heading home. We started talking. We talked about his family in Pennsylvania. I saw a different side of him. He didn't hound me about going out. He made me laugh; besides, he was good looking.

As time passes, I realize I want to get to know Keith better. I also understand he would never ask me out again. Who could blame him? I turned him down three times. I decide to ask him out. This was the eighties, but still I came from an era when women weren't assertive about such things. To make matters worse, I would have to catch him alone in the store, since that was the only time, I saw him.

Finally, I got up my nerve, "What are you doing this Saturday?"

"Not sure. Why? You need some help with the pump?"

I'm dying here. "No, my boys are with their dad this weekend. I was thinking about dinner and a movie."

Keith picked me up on Saturday. And so it began.

After seeing him several times. I introduced him to the boys. Acting like a big kid, Keith enjoyed taking them on the carnival rides, which terrified me. When I later signed them up for Little League, he came to practices and games without my asking. Eventually, he became their coach.

When the two-year waiting period ended, the courts granted my divorce. I made one last trip to Virginia Beach to sign the papers in the mediator's office. On the return trip, about thirty miles from home, my car broke down. I was wearing a lightweight red dress with matching espadrille wedges. Not exactly walking attire. No flats in the car. No cell phone. After I walked about five miles, a friend stopped and gave me a ride home. After the boys were in bed, Momma and I celebrated my freedom with Asti Spumante.

Keith and his brother purchased a home on Apple Mountain once they settled the insurance claim from the house they lost in the flood. Several months later, they lost it in a fire. Keith moved in with the boys and me. Along with him came his two dogs, Beau and Shane. Not long after, he proposed. I accepted.

We went to meet his family in Pennsylvania. Not knowing all the family history, I was anxious since I was a divorced woman with two children. Although we were in our thirties, Keith had never married. Even in the late eighties, being divorced was not as common as it is to-day. Turns out I worried about nothing; Keith's mom had two children from a previous marriage when she married his dad.

His family was very welcoming. Mom was more reserved than most of the family. Her conversational style was only somewhat warmer than an interrogation and had the same result. She had to know everything. Mom was almost always talking. She once told me, "When there's a lull in conversation, I feel I have to fill it".

His dad was different. When I first met him, he smiled at me as we backed up from a hug. "You have two choices. You can call me Colonel, or you can call me Dad."

I smiled back. "I think Dad will do."

Like me, he didn't mind companionable silence. We sat on the back porch of the cabin watching birds at the feeders. He put peanuts out so the blue jays and chipmunks would come to the porch to eat them.

In the 1986 World Series, the Mets beat the Red Sox. For me, it was fantastic. I fell in love with the Mets while in junior high. My math teacher would put on ball games during class. The Mets didn't take many divisional playoffs, but I loved them just the same. Now I could actually watch the Mets instead of following the box scores in the paper. Keith was a diehard Red Sox fan. To make matters worse, his mother was pulling for the Mets that year. The family joke goes that Keith nearly canceled the wedding because of that series.

Keith and I married in the Blackwell Methodist Church. I just wanted a small ceremony, but Keith and his family were eager to have the ceremony in the church. Everyone thought it was funny when I said I would not have the word "obey" in my vows. I stood my ground. Wedding vows are serious. I would not lie. I would not vow to obey.

Mom did most of the legwork since she was in the area. We exchanged long letters about what I wanted at the ceremony. She even got into it with a neighbor for picking roadside peonies for the church. Small, embroidered hearts edged in lace designated the family pews. My family and I made the food for our small reception.

Terry was my matron of honor. Jimmy and David walked me down the aisle. We were nearly an hour late starting the ceremony because I refused to go to the church until Momma was there. Keith's brother would walk back to the house to see if I'd heard from Momma. I sent word back to Keith that waiting for Momma was the only hold up. Dad fed me seven and sevens as I paced and looked out the window for my aunt's car. Momma and my aunt got lost driving up from Virginia but made finally it. The church was small, so only family members attended the service.

Nearly everyone from the village and surrounding area attended our reception on the flat behind the cabin. After the toasts, Keith's brothers tossed him into the Sucker hole. That seemed to be the signal for the party to begin. We spent our wedding night at a Williamsport hotel. After picking the boys up the next day, we headed back to Virginia.

Especially once we married, Keith and I had little time or money for date nights. Our alone time was often riding through the countryside in the truck while Momma watched the kids. We'd talk about where we'd like to live—not Front Royal and what we'd like to do. He was always telling stories about his family being stationed in Hawaii or Germany. Or when he lived in Utah or Florida. Riding down country roads takes me back to those early years.

Keith took me to an Elton John concert. He really prefers country music but took me because I had never gone to an Elton John concert, even though I bought all his records. My Audi overheated in the traffic jam that occurred as we neared the venue, but he got us there. All night he kept singing and smiling as I danced and sang my heart out. Later we went to Wolf Trap to see Three Dog Night. Again, we sang and danced in the aisles.

19

Grandmother's Attic

Grandmother's Attic was the embodiment of Momma's philosophy that multiple income streams led the way to financial security. People shooting pool were causing more trouble with the ABC board and patrons were getting rowdier. Momma's respiratory problems were getting worse. By spring, I was pregnant with Kenny. Neither of us was up to the hassle of dealing with it.

Once the pool table was out, we expanded the seating area for the snack bar. Using booths and shelving for room dividers, we created an area to feature depression glass, vintage clothing, and craft items made by Momma and me. Grandmother's Attic came to life. Eventually, we added a section for household items because people coming up for the weekend usually left something they needed behind at home.

We created a nursery in an extra-large closet in the hall near our bedroom. We had an old iron crib sandblasted. I painted it white and blue. Kenny arrived with no difficulties. He was born in the old Winchester Hospital. Keith brought me roses.

Loading Kenny into Momma's Buick, we scoured local flea markets and yard sales looking for forgotten treasures. In those days, people would just put out a "Yard Sale" sign. No advertising in the papers. No Facebook notices or Marketplace. Once we got to a sale, we'd all get out. Momma and I switching between checking the merchandise and keeping the Kenny in line.

At one sale run by an older lady, there were some things pulled out and put on tables in the driveway. We made several nice finds there, but we could see that she still had boxes stacked in the garage. Judging by the dust, they'd been there a while. For Momma, that was like Kmart having a blue light special.

"What have you got in the back of the garage there?" she asked.

"Don't rightly know. I haven't been all the way back there for 20 years or more."

Momma's eyes lit up a bit. "Mind if my daughter looks?"

"That's fine. Just don't hurt yourself."

"Sherry, climb up and check out those boxes."

There I go. Climbing in and amongst the boxes. I try to hide the fact that I'm afraid of finding a snake, spider, or something dead. I go through the boxes. "Momma, look at this."

As she gets closer, I show her the box of flat irons and another box with plates from the forties and fifties. "We don't have flat irons like this, and these dishes fill in the Homer Laughlin set I have."

Momma worked out a price, and we loaded up the Buick. She was always better at haggling than me. I'd look at the price and decide whether I could make a profit. If yes, then I'd buy it. Otherwise, I left it. If it was a big haul, Keith and I would come back later with his truck. After an outing, we'd pour over the reference books, clean up and tag our findings.

Grandmother's Attic also featured our handmade crafts. If we weren't searching for old glass, we were hunting for inexpensive supplies for our crafts. It started with an expansion of the Christmas ornaments Momma had made for several years. I made counted cross stitch ornaments. Eventually, I made several types of Christmas ornaments. I also specialized in lining baskets. Sometimes I sold just the lined baskets, but I'd usually have one or two filled with items for a last-minute baby shower or hostess gift.

In July, we would start making ornaments for sale in the shop and at juried craft shows in small towns like Middleburg. Juried craft shows brought in the most money but could be difficult. The application had to have pictures of your work and you had to demonstrate one of your crafts while you're at the sale. Of course, nothing could come from a kit. We made money at the shows, but it also brought customers to the store since we always took our business cards.

I was pregnant again at 33. In 1989, they termed this a high-risk geriatric pregnancy. Afraid of complications, my obstetrician ordered a lot of tests. He cautioned us babies born to mothers at my age had an increased chance of having Down's syndrome. Keith and I decided that no matter what, I would carry the baby to full term. All the testing was negative for any abnormalities, and we found we were having a baby girl.

As I did with my previous pregnancy, I continued working in the store, standing for long hours, lifting cases of beer to stock the coolers. At about six months into my pregnancy, I started having contractions. *This is too soon. What's going on?*

My obstetrician put me on bed rest with no lifting. Not even Kenny, who was just over a year old.

"How will I help support my children? I must work."

"You have two choices. Bed rest and have a healthy baby or work and lose the baby."

I cried in the parking lot, unsure how I could manage this change. Keith started doing his own laundry and doing more cooking. The older boys, at 8 and 10, began learning to do laundry and wash dishes. Momma still had the apartment next door, but was working as a nanny. She stopped by when she could. Often she cooked a big pot of soup while she visited and helped me clean the house.

A dark cloud was forming. Not like a hurricane. This was more personal. Right over my head. I wasn't sure about bringing up a daughter. The way for women was so fraught with dangers from so many sources. *How could I teach her to be a good, loving person and still protect herself? I had nightmares.*

I had thought all would be well once Sarah was born safely. My mood continued to plummet. It didn't help it that Kenny had reversed his sleep pattern and was awake most of the night. He and Sarah slept at opposite times. At least it was summer, and the older boys didn't need to be in school.

Keith got up at four in the morning to be at work at six. After work, he split wood to sell in the winter. Eventually, with the help of my pediatrician, Kenny got on a regular schedule.

We grew an extensive garden. I canned or froze what we didn't eat that summer. After some experimentation, I canned spaghetti sauce. Then I went to work canning peaches and green beans purchased from a roadside stand. I made jams. Also, I worked on items for the upcoming craft shows.

The cloud thinned out a little. I knew finances played a large part in my mood. I had to make more money. Keith was already working all the overtime he could, as well as selling wood. Momma sold the store. For a while, we kept Grandmother's Attic running. Sarah joined Kenny, Momma, and me on our jaunts to yard sales or craft stores. Depression glass was wildly popular then and reproductions were everywhere. It became harder to find authentic items. Craft items were being made overseas much more cheaply than we could make them. Ripples from the market spread out. The ripples made it clear. I needed to make a change.

I began making the first small steps in my quest to improve my mental health. I could acknowledge that I had experienced trauma, but recognized it didn't have to define me. Part of it for me was not allowing the trauma any power in my life. As I worked through this, I developed a mantra that helped me reduce the effect of the dreams. "You have no power. I have the power," Not that the dreams never occurred again, just that I could recognize them for what they were and move on without being devastated for days.

20

Beginning of a New Career

At first, I looked at positions related to my accounting degree. There weren't many opportunities in Front Royal. Childcare expenses made commuting to Manassas or Winchester economically unfeasible. Besides, helping Momma keep the books for the store made me realize I didn't enjoy accounting. I wanted to do something that mattered. I had always liked medicine and nursing.

While searching the want ads, I saw an ad from the local hospital. "Train to become a certified nursing assistant. Only $89 for a twelve-week course," the ad read. No guarantee of a job at the end, but I'd know if I could hack being a nurse.

Typical of me, I decided I was going to take the course before I talked to Keith. Before actually signing up, I told him what I was going to do. He felt I shouldn't have to work. His mother never worked outside the home. I grew up with a strong woman who always worked. I knew nothing else. Keith really couldn't work more than he was. I signed up for the course.

Training as a certified nursing assistant involved a lot of basics: taking blood pressures, weights, temperatures. After nine weeks of classroom work, we went to the bedside. We worked both in the hospital and in its attached long term care facility. For the first week, we partnered with an experienced certified nursing assistant. Most of the patients were alert, but there were a few that weren't. The bed baths weren't that difficult as they taught us how to maintain privacy, only uncovering the area we were washing. Sometimes turning a patient with mobility issues was difficult.

A kind older patient taught me to take a moment and put a hot washcloth on his face before shaving to reduce irritation and make shaving easier. By our last week, we held an eight-patient assignment. I passed the course.

A couple of months later, I took the written test and practicum for state certification. The written test was simple. I was anxious about performing care under the watchful eyes of the proctors who handed out cards which outlined our tasks. Some were simple: take full vital signs, transfer to wheelchair and transport to the dining room. I drew "take vital signs, give complete bed bath, change linens and set up for breakfast". Chatting with the "patient" as I provided care proved calming, and I later learned, earned extra points. I passed.

Of course, becoming a CNA wasn't the only thing happening in my life. The older boys played Little League, so there were games to go to and manage. I was still working. I slept a few hours here and there. To make matters worse, my personal cloud still hovered over me. The nightmares and flashbacks from my childhood continued. I was working through them but hadn't mastered them yet. Momma's health was worse. For a while, she lived with her sister in Nokesville. Then Momma moved into a house near her sister. I would go over to visit, help with the house or a project in the yard.

We did everything as a family. We ate dinner together every night. The younger children went to Little League games with us. We watched the Orioles play baseball at Memorial Stadium. Jimmy was involved in Math Counts and Odyssey of the Mind. Our vacations were visiting Keith's family. At the cabin, I'd cook Dad his favorite roast beef dinner with mashed potatoes and gravy.

The play Cats was big on Broadway. Jimmy's English class did a production using a couple of scenes from the play. Momma and I put his costume together. I learned to do the makeup for cat faces. Momma and Keith's parents joined us for the performance.

Six of us now crowded into our two-bedroom apartment. Kenny was still in his nursery and would soon outgrow his crib. Sarah's crib was in our bedroom. Keith and I talked about moving. We wanted to buy a house, but few of the places we looked at qualified for a VA loan. I just wanted to move so we could have more room, even if it meant renting again. With effort, I kept shoving all the stress away.

Just after Thanksgiving, Keith and I separated. I pulled the children out of school and moved us in with Momma in Nokesville. Jimmy and David had a room. Kenny and Sarah were in my room. We split Momma's sewing room to have a play area for the kids. I found a job at an assisted living facility in Manassas.

To be honest, Keith and I didn't talk about separating. I just moved me and the kids out. I was afraid because many of the men previously in my life were physically or verbally abusive to me or Momma. Nothing about Keith ever made me feel he would be abusive. But I was afraid he would convince me to change my mind.

I felt we didn't want the same things, but didn't really know how to get at what he truly wanted. At an early age, I learned how to live within myself and didn't know how to share deep thoughts and feelings. I kept them inside until they exploded. We talked more while separated than we had in several months. I learned that while we looked at things from different perspectives and had different ideas about planning, our core values and love for each other remained true. By the end of summer, we were back together and moved to a town house in Marshall. Although it took years, with Keith's patience, I learned to express my feelings *before* the explosion occurred.

Nursing still called to me. Not just the ability to make more money, although that was important, too. I remembered walking to the health department with Momma to get my vaccinations for school. Then there was Life magazine with its pictures of nurses caring for people in iron lungs because they couldn't breathe on their own after having polio.

Or the nurses who handed out the sugar cubes when I got my polio vaccine. All the books I read about public health advances in the United States centered on women, nurses. I wanted to be one of them.

I continued to work in Manassas. I took advantage of their generous tuition assistance program and enrolled at the community college to complete a few prerequisites for nursing school. Since I bought into the feminist concept that I could have it all, I was a scout leader for my daughter's daisy troop and started a T-ball team for Kenny and Sarah. David helped coach that team. As the younger kids moved up in Little League, Jimmy kept statistics for all the players. Eventually, Keith took over coaching for the T-ball team and I was manager/scorekeeper. Unless I was working, we still ate dinner as a family.

Finally, I applied to Shenandoah University's nursing program. I interviewed with the Dean of Nursing. A few weeks later, the letter arrived. Hands shaking, I opened the letter. Shenandoah accepted me for the fall semester. I danced around the kitchen.

For the first year of nursing school, I continued working in Manassas. I went down to four days a week. It kept me at full time so I wouldn't lose the tuition assistance. Classes Monday, Wednesday, Friday. Work Tuesday, Thursday, Friday, and every other weekend.

In between this, I went to Momma's for a few hours on my off weekend to help with whatever needed doing around the house. On one visit, I was helping transplant a holly tree and plant some new shrubs. Keith had found Momma a holly tree. Her plan was to move a holly growing into a fence and plant a small butterfly bush in its place. I would plant the holly from the fence down near a bench in the front yard. The new holly would go by the front porch. She couldn't do heavy work like digging

The new holly was easy to plant. Preparing the hole for the tree being moved away from the fence wasn't. The red clay was bone dry. I begin by digging a hole that was to be three feet deep and two feet wide. I pause for a minute.

"Momma, are you sure we can get that tree out of the fence without killing it? It looks awfully close to the fence to me."

"Sure, we can."

"Okay Momma. I'll keep digging."

After an hour of sweating, I finish digging the hole. We walk across the yard to the holly tree growing into the fence. I have to get through the hard clay and under the chain-link fence to the root ball of the holly tree. Momma watches as I dig.

"Sherry, I think you're right. Getting this tree out will cut major roots. Guess the butterfly bush will have to go down by the bench." She strokes my shoulder. "Sorry baby."

"It's okay Momma. How about putting on some coffee while I finish up?"

When we got the tools put away, Momma and I sat on the front porch to drink our coffee and watch Kenny and Sarah ride down the hill on their train made from tying Momma's small, wheeled garden seat to the back of a tricycle. We both laughed about digging a three-foot hole for a plant in a gallon container.

In my second semester of nursing school, we had to take a "Math Calculations for Nurses" course. Basic algebra for dose calculations. Stuff I knew. I kept flubbing the tests. In talking with my professor, we uncovered my anxiety. She made a referral to the therapist at the school's health center. Where I was introduced me to guided imagery, a relaxation technique that has served me well once I learned to apply it. It took years for me to master the technique.

Momma bought me self-help books from Serve, like Richard Carlson's *Don't Sweat the Small* Stuff. I had trouble determining *what was the small stuff. In my mind, there was no small stuff.* There were so many things I needed to be or do: be a good mother and wife, be a good daughter, do well in school, so well in my job to keep the paycheck, and have a clean home. Professors counseled my to stop working, but could offer no alternative income sources. So, my merry-go-round continued,

Although I had regular childcare, Momma took care of Kenny and Sarah if their regular sitter wasn't available, or Jimmy had a Math Counts competition. This also gave Jimmy and David some free time since they regularly helped with their younger siblings. Kenny often tagged at David's heels for pickup basketball and Jimmy taught multiplication while supervising bath time. When they were with her, Momma frequently took Kenny and Sarah to the local hospital thrift store, where she volunteered. The kids played in the toy section while Momma sorted items for the shop. The ladies running the shop appreciated Momma's knowledge of old glass and other vintage items as it helped them price items accordingly.

Momma ran a perpetual yard sale from her garage. Most of the items she offered were leftover stock from Grandmother's Attic. All the kids would help her set up. Kenny and Sarah, in particular, loved to be there on yard sale days. Momma always let each kid set up a small area of their own and keep the proceeds from their sale. She taught all of them about pricing and merchandising. "Price it so that you make money but not so high no one will buy it." "Set it up nice. So, it looks good and catches the eye."

She loved being a grandmother. Not just with things, but with her time. Helping with craft projects or baking little bunny cakes for Easter. Going to school and sporting events when we lived in the same area. She once made a small fire in her side yard so Kenny and Sarah could roast marshmallows with her.

These were also the years of what I call magical Christmases. All the children were home. We started decorating the Saturday after Thanksgiving. The six of us piled into the van. We rode around to the different Christmas tree stands in the area, searching for the perfect tree. In the end, we bought the tree from the Boy Scouts. Keith would get the tree up in the stand and string the lights. He and I always had a running debate about how many lights the tree needed. I always wanted more.

As the kids and I hung the ornaments, I told them how Momma made the snowman ornaments from small socks. One for each of us.

Or how the ceramic ones were free with a tank of gas at 7-11. In fact, Momma and I made nearly all the ornaments on the tree, so there were lots of stories. Later, we'd all string popcorn garlands to finish out the tree. Until I started nursing school, we each made a new group of ornaments every year. For me, Christmas was about being with family and decorating.

Celebrating began on Christmas Eve at Momma's. She'd have home-made vegetable soup and cornbread ready. After dinner, we exchanged gifts. The children watched a Christmas special while we cleaned up.

The kids always woke up early on Christmas Day---especially Sarah. We opened presents and then had a big country breakfast. Often, Jimmy and David would celebrate Christmas with Jim later that day. When he was on shore duty, they spent most of the school holiday with him. During the week between Christmas and New Year's Eve, we would make a trip to Baltimore to have Christmas with Keith's family.

At Shenandoah University, all second-year nursing classes had to be taken in a specific order. I would have to be in class four days a week. I left the assisted living facility and took a job in home health. It was hard to leave. Polly, the RN in charge, had been such a positive force, always collaborating with me to create a schedule that didn't interfere with school.

After a few typical assignments that had me working in different homes, I got lucky. A lady needed round-the-clock care. She had a stroke several years before as well as dementia. The widow of a prominent government official, Ella, lived outside a small town near Marshall. Ella and I got on well. Soon, her conservators had me booked for every shift I was available.

The easiest home health job ever. Ella slept late, until 11 in the morning, and then was asleep by seven. Her breakfast was fresh fruit, a pastry and coffee. A local restaurant Ella used to frequent catered and delivered her meals daily. While Ella slept, I did some light housework, a couple of loads of laundry, and studied. After breakfast, we would go on the deck and watch the Canadian geese and deer she fed. I would read the Washington Post to her or set up the TV for PBS. Then microwave dinner, help Ella get ready for bed and study.

Disaster struck during the second semester. My van's engine went. This time there was nothing Keith could do. He'd kept it running much longer than it should have. While we were scrambling around trying to figure out how to come up with a vehicle for me, Keith's dad offered his truck. "Sherry's got to finish now or else wait a year. Come up and get my truck. We can live with one car a few months 'til she graduates." On a weekend, Momma watched the kids while Keith and I drove up to Pennsylvania for the truck. It had jump seats, so I could get the younger kids around.

Momma was in and out of the hospital twice during that semester. Her asthma kept flaring and then she would get pneumonia. While she was in the hospital, I deep cleaned everything... removing all dust. This was tough, since she displayed her multiple collections on open shelving. I got her crafting supplies into containers that would keep them dust free and installed HEPA filters in her HVAC system.

Keith's parents moved to Maryland. Mom had had enough of the Pennsylvania weather and lifestyle. Keeping up with the cabin was getting to be too much for them. Dad was unhappy about being away from Blackwell. He made frequent trips back to Pennsylvania. We would join him when our crazy schedules permitted.

The moment I'd worked for came. Graduation. Momma and Keith's parents were there, as were Keith and the kids. I was so proud and happy. I graduated with honors. Jimmy was entering college in the fall. David graduated from high school in June. In July, I passed my boards.

Families make their own traditions, weaving them onto the ones handed down from previous generations. When the children were young, we spent a lot of our family time on a ball field. Keith and I both loved baseball. We loved family. Our family has no "steps" just Dad, Mom, brothers, and sister. There is a ten-year space between the two groups of children.

Once the kids showed an interest, we saw sports as a bridge between the age differences. Since everyone is not athletic, we also played board games as a family. Even in their young adulthood, we would gather to watch the World Series, Super Bowl, or play games. With everyone spread out geographically, we often call or text about great plays as we watch the same game in our individual homes. Now we play Chutes n Ladders or Candyland with our five-year-old grandson. Both he and our three-year-old granddaughter often sit beside me to watch a baseball game.

21

The Making of a Nurse

I found a 3pm to 11pm position at the continuing care center (CCC) in Marshall. There was a small skilled unit, a special needs unit, as well as an assisted living unit. I was so excited about having my first nursing job. I'd be making $13.00 an hour. That was almost double what I made as a CNA. The facility was less than ten minutes from home.

Residents of a CCC expect to live there forever. Insurance covered some care, but primarily it was a private pay facility. The largest unit was independent/assisted living. There was a small skilled nursing unit and a special needs unit. Most residents had been doctors or some big wig in government. Furniture and other items from home filled their living areas.

Initially, I worked on the skilled unit. One certified nursing assistant helped with the care of 10 residents. Mostly I hung IV antibiotics and fluids. There was a small amount of wound care involved. One lady had a stroke several years ago and now had a feeding tube. She could not communicate or provide any self-care. I learned to do MDSs, a complicated assessment that determines a facility's payment for care provided to an individual.

Most of the doctors rounding on the unit were pretty collaborative. My favorites were the ones who taught without being patronizing. Then there was the charting on every resident. Not just how they did that shift, but details to justify their need for skilled care. In those days, charting was all handwritten. Day shift wrote in blue; evening shift wrote in green and night shift wrote in red. We transcribed orders in black. That changed to all black in a couple of years.

I was the only nurse working the unit and the only RN in the building, such responsibility for a newly licensed nurse. There were nurses working the other units. One, Bob, was very helpful when I wasn't sure about a procedure or orders. He was a licensed practical nurse (LPN) and had practiced in the Air Force. Unlike some, he didn't bother with the RN versus LPN nonsense and would give straight forward help when needed. I learned a great deal of practical bedside knowledge from him.

If someone died in the facility, an RN had to pronounce them dead. It's really a simple matter of listening to the heart and noting the absence of pulse and respirations. When I had to do this the first time, it was for one of Bob's patients. He stayed around, noting times for me. After I made the pronouncement, Bob and I headed back to the nurses' station.

"Were you having trouble hearing or something?"

"No. I was just struggling with the concept of pronouncing someone dead. I mean..."

"Yeah, I get it. Even though it's not a code, you say this is the end and you get a similar feeling."

"Exactly. I'll fill out the paperwork and call the doctor. Then I'll call the family."

"I've got a good a good relationship with the family. They've been expecting this, so I'll call them."

Other nurses carried some resentments. They considered my position with a lower census a cushy job. Most of the LPNs had the experience and could fill the position. Federal regulation required that an RN be present in the skilled unit on all three shifts to bill for Medicare.

The evening shift was hard on me and my family. I had a hard time winding down after getting home. Keith got up early for work and I had to get the children up for school. One evening, Bob stopped by to see if I wanted to take a break.

"Sherry, are you okay? You look a little pale."

"I'm okay. Just my stomach. I had an ulcer once. Feels like it's starting up again."

"You better get it checked out."

A trip to the doctor yielded a prescription for Pepcid. He encouraged me to reduce my stress. Everyone says the same thing, but no one can tell me how to do it. I have responsibilities. *There is no small stuff.*

The special needs unit was home to residents who could no longer care for themselves because of a cognitive impairment. Certified nursing assistants (CNAs) provided help with dressing, eating, and toileting. A nurse passed medications and helped the CNAs when they could. The rest of the time, the residents wandered around the closed unit. Dignity was hard to find.

After working on the skilled unit for about six months, the director of nursing offered me a position as lead RN on the special needs unit. This would be a day shift position. Staff would receive additional training focused on caring for with residents with dementia. Promoting dignity would be our cornerstone.

Residents found their rooms by looking for a photograph beside their door. Family members helped set this up by finding a picture the resident recognized from their past. It might be their wedding photograph or one of their young children. We held classes for family members to help them understand how to best interact with their loved ones as their dementia progressed. Because they helped design the program, all staff members were invested in its success.

We had an after-school program which allowed staff members' children to be Junior volunteers. Children got off the school bus off at the front door. They read to residents, sang with them, or did an arts and crafts project. A highlight of the year was a Christmas program. Most of the residents had trouble communicating verbally. Because it was a long-term memory, most could remember words to songs they sang when they were younger.

In the program, residents sang Christmas carols with the children as another resident accompanied them on the piano. Of all the jobs I've had in nursing, this is high on my list of favorites. They promoted me to the assistant director of nursing role at this facility. I got my first cell phone. It truly was a small brick. Nothing like our smart phones today.

Of course, while I'm figuring out this nursing business, life outside nursing continues. Dad had fallen while he was up at the cabin. He fractured his hip and lay in the yard several hours before a neighbor saw him and called an ambulance. Dad's hospital stay was brief. After a short rehab stint, he was back in Maryland. Blood clots in his leg prolonged his recovery.

Jimmy returned from Virginia Tech. He had a job and now lived with a roommate. David moved to Illinois to live with his dad. There was a hole I struggled to fill with both older boys gone. *How can I protect you when you're far away? How will I know if you're sick or hungry?* I knew they couldn't stay home forever, and, in fact, I had raised them to be independent. Still, I worried about taking care of everyone.

I remembered a television program I watched just before Jimmy graduated high school. The commentator talked about children leaving home for college. He encouraged parents to take heart and see their children as ships carrying their flag to new worlds. He reassured us that the ships would come back to port. I held fast to that hope.

Martin moved to Texas. After several months, Momma and I flew down to attend his wedding. We attended the rehearsal dinner and a couple of family events. Everyone was gracious.

There were a lot of family discussions about Dad not going to the cabin without someone. Since Mom did not want to go back as often as Dad did, it became a bone of contention. The family would all go up at the beginning of spring to open the cabin for the season. On long week-end holidays, Keith and I would drive up with the kids so Dad could spend time in Blackwell. Dad could never spend enough time there.

The Comstock family started trying to find a solution that would appease both Dad and Mom. None of Keith's siblings could drop their lives and go live in Blackwell. After much discussion among ourselves and our respective families, Keith and I decided to the move to Blackwell full time.

Blackwell was a small community, offering lots of outdoor experiences. In contrast, the townhouse community in Marshall was changing. Small-time drug dealers started hanging around the playground. Fights among kids were happening more frequently. My heart froze as I thought about moving away from Momma. She still drove and made her own appointments, of course. Aunt BJ was nearby. But no one would help take care of her flowers. Momma encouraged me to do the best for my family.

The actual move took several months. Kenny and Sarah had to finish their school year and Little League seasons. Keith and I needed to find employment. Initially, I applied for director or assistant director of nursing positions. Without receiving a positive response by March, I applied to the hospital in Wellsboro. From my time as a student nurse, I knew I didn't like hospital nursing; the patients weren't there long enough. But I thought I could work in the hospital a year before returning to administration in long term care. It would hone my bedside skills and give me time to find the right facility. There's a prevailing attitude in nursing that you must have at least a short period of medical-surgical nursing on your resume to be considered a proper nurse. To some extent, they're right; it all depends upon your area of specialization and marketability, should you decide to change jobs.

It took a few weeks to set up an interview with the hospital. Dad met us at the cabin. It was bitterly cold. The weather forecast called for snow. My winter coat purchased for Virginia weather did little to stop the biting wind. I felt the interview went well. Although we discussed when I would move to the area, I didn't receive an offer.

We planned to go home on Saturday. Snow began falling in the middle of the night. Keith was very experienced driving in the snow, so we headed out after breakfast. Dad would stay until the weather cleared.

Freezing rain joined the snow, making the roads treacherous. Keith kept the van on the road with a lot of difficulty. Everyone was quiet so he could concentrate on driving. At the turkey ranch, the van fishtailed ever so slightly. The fat snowflakes fell so thickly we could barely see a car length ahead. People abandoned cars and left them at odd angles along the side of the highway.

"Honey, better call work and then Dad while you have cell service. I don't think we can make it up this hill. I can turn around right up the road."

"Hey Mindy, sorry to bother you on the weekend, but the weather has turned rotten here. I'm not sure I will be at work on Monday. It depends on how quickly they can clear the roads. I'll keep you posted."

"Don't worry about getting in here on Monday. You guys just stay safe."

Dad was relieved when I told him we were turning around. "Just take your time."

. Not having planned to stay longer than Saturday morning, we all troop across the road to the hotel for dinner. Nice, pleasant company as the owner and Dad reminisce about the summer and days gone by. Looking out the window at the snow made me shiver and reach for a sweater.

Within a few days of returning to Marshall, I received a job offer from the hospital in Wellsboro, understanding that I would start in July. Now the real flurry of activity began as I collected boxes and began packing. In those days, we collected boxes from grocery stores or work, no running to Lowes to buy boxes for moving. Time flew by. Kenny and Sarah finished up school. Their Little League season was winding down.

Historically, it was a hard time for LPN's, most of them had worked in hospitals and were proficient in many of the skills I learned in nursing school. However, in response to a push from nurse educators, regulators and nurse associations, hospitals were requiring a bachelor's degree in nursing or at least entry into a bachelor's program for entry level nursing positions. Since Florence Nightingale's era, nursing has struggled to be seen as a profession. Hospital based diploma programs were ending, nurses with two-year degrees were being pushed to get their masters or even doctorate degree. This left most LPNs working in assisted living facilities or long-term care and the LPN's thought this wasted their skills. It's a problem that still concerns the nursing profession today.

22

Pennsylvania--Land of Frozen Water

Blackwell sits in a valley along Pennsylvania's Grand Canyon. State land surrounds the village and large creeks curve around three of its sides. Oak, cottonwood, and pine trees cover the mountains as they carve out their space among large areas of exposed rock. Its raw natural beauty is breathtaking. Even winter snows bring a stark beauty to the mountains surrounding the village.

Morris is about 10 minutes away from Blackwell. Besides a cluster of homes, Morris has a general store, a couple of bars, churches, a restaurant, and the volunteer fire and rescue department. Each bar serves at least some food to keep it within regulation. When you reach the Morris township line, you pick up cell phone service.

Morris has two big events: Rattlesnake Round Up in the summer and Old Home Days in the fall. I was accustomed to being minutes from a grocery store. In Virginia, where were always craft fairs and estate sales to go to that involved collectibles and antiques, not farm equipment and tractor pulls.

Turning left at Morris' second stop sign, a thirty-minute drive takes you to the nearest grocery store in Wellsboro. If you continue for another half hour, you reach Walmart in Mansfield. Turning right at that stop in Morris, a 45-minute drive takes you to Kenny and Sarah's school in Liberty. When we moved in, the village's census rose to 28. The hotel across the street has a new owner and caters to tourists. The church Keith and I were married in no longer holds regular services. There was talk that they would convert the railroad tracks to hiking trails.

Despite the isolation and differences in the region, I was excited about the prospect of living in Blackwell. We would help Keith's parents and we would live in a house. Black walnut trees lined the back yard or "the flat" as we called it. Several of them were too large to get my arms around. The cabin was originally Keith's grandmother's home.

In the 1940s, the railroad floated the rectangular core of the building down the creek. There was a tannery in Blackwell and a railroad stop then. Over the years, the house sprouted additions to accommodate differing needs. In its final evolution, the cabin became a split level with a walkout basement and two bonus rooms over the garage. There was a deck leading out from upstairs to the back porch. The family called the bonus rooms over the garage the Pest Hole because that's where the children hung out. Throughout Keith's childhood as an Army brat, it was the place they returned to and called home. Oh yeah, no central air or heat. No internet service.

By the end of June, I finished my last shifts at the CCC. Momma had us over for dinner the night before we headed up to Blackwell. I knew we made the right decision. But each decision has positive and negative aspects. Early the next morning, Keith, the kids, and I headed out. We had filled my van and Keith's truck with the first load. It was nice that the necessities were already in the cabin. Even though it meant moving things around until I understood what Mom wanted to do with the things she left behind.

Once we unloaded, Kenny and Sarah claimed their rooms and headed outside to explore. I had decided that the Pest Hole, once revamped, would be excellent for the guest area. I wanted to make it special and a bit more private—particularly when Dad and Mom came to visit. Keith hooked up the washer and dryer.

There wasn't much unpacking that night as we headed into Wellsboro to pick up groceries. Mostly, I bought milk, coffee, cereal, tuna, and other things for sandwiches. I'd be working a 3 pm to 11pm shift and for a couple of weeks I would be on my own, as both Kenny and Sarah had Little League playoffs to complete.

I'd never been away from them longer than overnight when they had a sleepover at Momma's. I hugged them both tightly, "Call me when you get home"

"We will, Momma," they both promised.

"I'll call you honey," as Keith gave me a last hug.

I fought back tears, watching Keith and the kids drive off to Virginia. Once they were out of sight around the curve, I grabbed some coffee and sat on the back porch. I could hear all the birds, but no traffic, no neighbors. It was nice. But it would take a while to get used to the quiet. My thoughts turned to making a home here and hoping that Momma's health didn't take a downward turn soon. Of course, I couldn't stop there. Worries about all my children plagued me.

To combat my anxieties, I unpacked, trying to work our things in with those already there. Thoughts of Mom's inspections were always in the back of my mind. To be honest, she never blamed me if the house was messy. Mom felt I had a lot on my plate and would fuss with Keith and the kids about helping more. Still, I was a product of my times. I felt responsible. It made me feel that somehow, I was lacking. Besides, she had always maintained the cabin so well. I got my uniforms unpacked and everything ready for work the next day. *If I get tired enough, I won't be able to think about things.* Exhausted, I fell asleep on the couch.

Caring for my patients and giving IV push medications for the LPNs working alongside me or maintaining their patients' central lines kept me busy. I learned to hang blood and do surgical wound care. It wasn't too bad unless there were a lot of admissions.

The hospital census was falling, so as the nurse last hired to the med-surg unit, I had to be oriented and then float to the pediatric unit. I loathed it. Shifting gears from treating adults to treating children was mind-boggling. Vital signs were different. Medications and dosing were different. As a student nurse, I knew I never wanted to work with children. To be frank, any babies stayed there only long enough to be transferred to a larger hospital. Still, I honed my nursing skills, became more efficient and tried to enjoy my work.

Sarah came up first. Her softball team took first place. Kenny's baseball playoffs took longer. Keith and I had promised the kids we would get a dog once we were more settled. When I had a day off, Sarah and I would go to the shelter in Wellsboro to see if there were any puppies for adoption. On our third visit, we adopted Champ. Or more accurately, he adopted us as he tumbled off the pile of his siblings and walked toward us.

Champ was a mutt. His tail curled up over his back most of the time. He followed Kenny and Sarah everywhere until they crossed a bridge or got in the water. Champ never liked bridges or water. He was very protective without being aggressive. One of our summer neighbors would fix him his own breakfast plate and leave it on their back steps for him to eat as he made his rounds of the neighborhood.

Once Kenny's baseball playoffs were complete, he and Keith joined us at the cabin. Keith found work clearing lines with a company. Not the tree work he enjoyed, but it was work. Keith was a certified arborist and was more accustomed to trimming trees to remove diseased portions or promote beauty and growth. Line clearing always left trees looking butchered, as the focus was on keeping limbs off a power line and clearing as much line as you could you in a day.

I spent every minute I wasn't at the hospital, organizing the house, or working in the yard. I finally had the Pest Hole area converted to guest rooms. For the upstairs portion, I made and hung curtains. I incorporated many of Mom's pieces into the décor. In the Pest Hole's lower level, I tucked a camp bed under the long window and set it up as a couch. I coordinated the linens for the bunk beds and the twin bed for Dad. Valances were up over the mini blinds. I couldn't wait for Dad and Mom to see them. I didn't have to wait long for Dad to make the trip.

"Sherry, the Pest Hole looks good. I appreciate you trying to make Mom comfortable, but I think she would be more comfortable in her old room."

"Okay, I'll get things changed back."

That was the hard part of living in the cabin. It was still the Comstock family home, and everyone always commented on any changes we made along the way. Mostly, everyone was positive, but not always.

I began working in the yard, expanding flower beds. With so much slate around, I terraced the hill which crested at the back porch. Momma was having trouble keeping up with her flowers, so I brought many of them to Pennsylvania. Later, clients would decide to make a change within their yard and Keith would bring home their discards for me to incorporate into the flower beds. Compared to the red clay I was used to, the black soil at the cabin was like planting in pure fertilizer. If they survived the cold, plants grew like wild.

Near the end of September, I received a call from a small community hospital I had applied to prior to moving. They were looking for a director of nursing for their extended care unit. I didn't enjoy working at the Wellsboro hospital. They were still floating me to pediatrics. And if the hospital census was low and there were no pediatric patients, I often sat at work for an hour and then had to go home. For Keith and me, it was a straightforward decision to at least interview and check it out.

The interview process had three parts. First with the administrator. Second, with department heads and key members from the extended care unit. Finally, a luncheon interview with the doctors and department heads from the hospital. The first two parts went well, and we set the final interview up for Friday.

Keith's parents were in town. They were both pleased with the way things were developing in the cabin and yard. Mom and Dad were very excited about the interview.

The hospital was an hour and a half from Blackwell. The route ran over some narrow back mountain roads. The interview went well. Lunch was excellent. The head of the hospital's dietary department was a chef. While the administrator and I toured the building, everyone else from the luncheon made their decisions. Before I left, I accepted the offer to start in October. I was on top of the world. Everything was coming together. The house. The yard. A position I wanted. More money.

After some discussion, Dad and Mom changed their plans. They would go back to Belair on Monday so they could take Keith and me to dinner on Saturday. We never got to dinner.

The next day, Dad woke up not feeling well. He hadn't felt a hundred percent since he fractured his hip several months ago. He was feeling weak, so I helped him into the bathroom and back to his recliner. Dad became unresponsive, even to a sternal rub. Another extra hard rub on the chest brought Dad around enough so he could focus on my face for a moment. Keith called the paramedics. Mom sat beside him, holding his hand, talking to him softly. The paramedics took him to in the Wellsboro hospital. Later, the doctors transferred him to the hospital in Williamsport. We lost him on October 13, 2000.

Dad planned for his body to be donated to a medical school. Keith's brothers organized Dad's memorial out back on the flat under a large tent. It was surreal. One minute we're getting ready to celebrate my promotion and the next we're celebrating Dad's life. His gun salute echoed through the valley.

Prior to 2000 arriving, everyone was afraid that there would be a major crash of the internet and computer programs because the year ended in 00. After spending a lot of money, it came down to everyone adopting the use four numbers instead of two to indicate a year. They avoided the crisis. This is a simplification, of course. Still, it's the simple stuff that marks our lives. Four digits to indicate a year kept the computer systems going, but losing a single man certainly changed the course of a family's future in so many ways.

23

First Winter

Arriving home after my first day at the extended care center, I came home to a cake. Keith and the kids made and decorated it to congratulate me on the new position. Kenny's childhood bear wore my graduation cap and honor cord. We played board games and watched a movie before the kids went to bed. Keith and I talked about how schedules would change as I started this new venture.

Fortunately, the school bus stopped right at the end of our driveway. I left the house at seven thirty every morning just as the bus picked up the kids. I rarely got home before six or seven in the evening. After dinner, there was always work in my briefcase.

Within a few months, we moved all the residents of the skilled unit onto two wings. The consolidation made it easier for staff to provide care and reduced the overall number of people needed to staff the unit. I then moved my office from the ground floor up to the second floor.

We converted two adjoining patient rooms on the closed wing to an office and conference room. The conference room allowed me to hold in-services and staff meetings without the conflicts that often arose if I used the hospital conference room. Also, I was closer to the residents and nurses. It simplified my daily rounding of each unit. At first, the decision was not popular with some department heads but paid off in the end, as family members and nurses would stop in for coffee and an impromptu visit. It gave me a chance to get to know them.

Winter came quickly. Snow and ice. Treacherous roads. At first, Keith would drive me to work and come back to pick me up. He never complained about spending the better part of his day driving. Finally, I got tough with myself and began driving in the snow. I always carried emergency supplies in the car to include heavy coveralls and boots. I also carried two cell phones, one personal and one work phone. There was no service while I was on the mountain. I called home before I started over the mountain when the weather was bad since so Keith could approximate my location should I run into trouble.

One Sunday, Keith, Kenny, and Sarah were sledding in a field off a back road. I never liked snow and stayed warm at home with hot chocolate on the ready. We already had six inches of snow and the creek had mostly frozen over. The weather forecast called for a nor'easter. It would bring another eight inches of snow, at least. Going to work Monday would be risky. I packed a suitcase for two or three days and headed out after everyone was home. This was not a new procedure. I had frequently done the same in Virginia when we had heavy snows.

During the storm, I often covered a CNA position because the LPNs could pass medications faster than I could. I scheduled myself so that I could assist on each shift as needs arose. We rolled a hospital bed into my office to give me some privacy when I slept. It was three days before the road over the mountain was clear enough for me to drive home and staffing was at acceptable levels. Those three days were probably the best morale booster for the nursing team. But man, was I glad to get home.

One of the hardest parts of this position was, besides being responsible for the SNF nursing department, I was the liaison between the hospital and the SNF. There were so many committees, meetings, family activities and trainings. All the nursing department heads were all overwhelmed. The hospital administrator introduced the nursing department heads to Steven Covey's concepts of time management. I was already using a planner. However, the concept of managing events was inspiring. After all, as Covey said, we cannot control time. I bought into it hook, line and sinker. Events were color coded, and I had only one calendar. Now I can manage my stress better. Or so I foolishly thought.

During winter, Keith's work shut down. Unlike his company in Virginia, which did snow removal during the winter, here they laid everyone off. We hadn't been in Pennsylvania long enough for him to draw unemployment. Thankfully, the cost of living was a lot less.

The decision to move my office up to the unit was not an easy one. It moved me away from some other administrative people but no further away from my administrator, as she was in the hospital, a separate building. In most cases, I feel administrators and directors of nursing should be physically closer in a building. This leads to more impromptu communication. As an outsider, I already had enough hurdles to jump. Bringing me closer to my staff proved helpful. The meeting room next door proved to be an excellent place for state surveyors.

Spring Into Summer

I started looking for forsythia in March. When I was eight, I realized forsythia, with its bright yellow bells on bare stalks, were among the first flowers to bloom in the spring. Ever since then, I eagerly look for them as the harbinger of spring.

The forsythia bush near the Babs Creek bridge finally began budding at the beginning of April. Today I wore a heavy sweatshirt as I raked leaves from the flower beds. It had snowed a couple of days ago, on the 10th, my birthday. It was really just a flurry, but I took it as a personal affront. Today was sunny but cold. I didn't want to waste any sunny days.

"Sherry, you aren't trying to plant yet, are you?" My next-door neighbor called out as she crossed the yard.

"No, not yet. Just thought I'd get the beds cleaned out some."

"You can probably plant by the middle of the month. More than likely in May to be safe."

As the weather got warmer, Kenny, Sarah, and I took my van up the mountain to gather the slate. I park on the shoulder. We start by picking up slate that had fallen to the shoulder. Kenny, always looking for adventure, begins climbing up the hill. The middle of the hill is slightly concave, and you can't see the top while you are climbing. My heart's in my throat. *What if he falls and breaks a leg or gets a concussion?*

"Kenny, get down from there."

"I'm okay Momma. You and Sarah back up and I'll toss it down."

Sarah and I wait for a few minutes. I try not to watch Kenny so intently. My protective side wars with the side that knows he needs to be independent and press his limits. Sarah grabs my arm as Kenny makes it nearly to the top of the hill.

"Momma, look up top. There's a snake."

"Kenny, get down. There's a snake right over your head," Sarah and I are both screaming now. "Get down here."

Nonchalantly, Kenny climbs back down and looks up once he's on the ground. The snake is coiled, shaking its rattles, and looking for the source of disruption on its sunny ledge. We put a few more pieces of slate into the van and head home. I couldn't handle being near that snake. Snake sightings would become more commonplace, and I'd eventually learn not "run for the hills" every time I saw one.

Spring also brought the ladybug invasion. These were not the cute little red insects with black dots. These were orange and swarmed like bees. Like many older homes, the areas around our windows didn't fit tightly. I would open curtains to find a horde of ladybugs huddled in the corners. As a defense mechanism, they secret a pungent odor when threatened. I would spray and then vacuum them up. You had to throw the vacuum cleaner bag away to avoid having the entire house smell like dead ladybugs. As we got the house sealed up better, the horde would get trapped between the window glass and screen. More vacuuming. They still smelled terrible.

We spent a lot of time on the back porch. It was the ideal relaxing place. Shade from the walnut trees lining the flat kept you cool. Besides feeding birds, we put out peanuts for the chipmunks who wound their burrows through the terraces of my flower beds. They would pop up to the porch, grab a peanut, disappear into the flowers, and turn up about 20 feet away to eat their prize. Sometimes another chipmunk would ambush the one popping out into the yard, and a fight would break out.

During a recent visit, Sarah reminded me of the time a chipmunk made its way inside. They found it up in the Pest Hole. Laughing hysterically, they tried to herd it back down the stairs and into the garage. Hearing the ruckus, I stuck my head into the stairwell and peered into the room. Apparently herding wasn't working so, they were trying to catch it by covering it with a small trash can. Sarah's trying to scare the chipmunk toward the trash can Kenny's holding. There was a swoosh and a miss. Then, like a scene in a cartoon, Sarah is running in place, trying not to step on the chipmunk darting around between her feet. Kenny makes a swoop with the trash can, and after missing, simply rolls over, laughing uncontrollably. Sarah drops beside Kenny and laughs just as hard. The chipmunk took this opportunity to escape down the stairs and out of the garage.

By the fourth of July, the yard was looking good. Keith grilled. I made potato salad and baked beans. My potato salad is different from the northern style, just potatoes, mayo, dill pickles, boiled eggs, and a hint of mustard. The kids ran about with their friends. Adults hung out and had a few drinks. After dark, there were fireworks down by the creek. We would do it again in September as our summer friends closed their cabins for winter.

25

Winter to Spring

Life really got interesting as Kenny began junior high. Sarah's friend Catherine moved to Lewisburg, and we often split the distance with her parents so the girls could stay connected. Kenny played basketball for the school's JV team. I often left work a little early to drive two hours to watch him play. Once home and after dinner, I worked on policy revisions. Many of the policies in place were more appropriate for the hospital than a SNF. I also wrote policies to cover changes we made within extended care.

I was reviewing policies with my nursing administrative staff when the executive assistant stuck her head in the door. "Turn on the TV. You've got to see what's happening in New York. They've bombed the World Trade Center."

Turning on the TV, we watch a replay of the World Trade Center's collapse after being struck by planes, hear about the attack on the Pentagon and the crash of Flight 93 in Somerset County. Somerset County is only 180 miles from Blackwell. Watching the scene unfold empties my lungs like a punch to the belly. Gaining our composure, we call our families and then brainstorm ways to send supplies to hospitals in New York.

It took a while for us to reach Jimmy. He was working in Arlington. His route to work took him close to the Pentagon. Fortunately, he was already at work during the attack. He and his friends were safe. Nothing was happening near Chicago, so David was safe.

For a while, I feared events would draw the country into a horrific war. In all-out war, the Army would draft my older sons. Keith and I worried about this for many months. In the end, things returned to normal. Although Homeland Security and terror alerts would forever change how we traveled.

The hours of driving, working, and keeping up with the family were taking its toll. Following a successful state inspection at work, I was having even more trouble with stress. My blood pressure, which had always been low, was climbing into the "not healthy range". I couldn't sleep.

I'm early for a meeting with my administrator. "Good morning, Dana." I pause near the door as she's busy at her computer.

"Good morning, Sherry. How are things going with the policy revisions?" Looking up from her keyboard, she asks, "Are you, okay? You look a little gray? Here, sit down. Let me check your blood pressure."

"I'm fine. Just didn't sleep well last night. I'm a little tired."

"168/101. Let's go down to the ED. I don't want you having a heart attack or a stroke."

With a bit more coaxing, I followed her downstairs. My blood pressure was still elevated. After reviewing lab results, the doctor admitted me for observation, since he felt I was having a cardiac event. Once the nurses completed the admission process, I fell asleep.

I woke up to find Keith and the kids at my beside.

"I'm going to be fine. The doctor just wants to be careful. If my labs later show nothing abnormal, I'll be home tomorrow."

The doctor admonished me for working so much and staying so stressed out. He also gave me a prescription for Paxil. While commonly prescribed for depression, it can reduce anxiety. I took it for a while but didn't like the way it made me feel, or rather, not feel. So, I stopped taking it. I resolved to do more of the things I liked to do.

Fortunately, it was spring. Working in a flower bed for me is like taking a dose of Valium. It's the next best thing to being on the beach.

I can forget about everything for at least for a little while when I've got my hands in dirt. There was always something to do in the garden. It's a bit like having an old cozy family quilt in my landscape since I've always planted flowers that remind me of special people in my life. I also like for the flower beds to provide a natural habitat for birds and butterflies.

This year, Keith took out an old section of decking and I worked to extend the flower garden around the corner of the porch. Blacked-eyed susans moved from other places in the yard, filled the top tier of the terrace and showed over the porch railing. Their yellow petals form around a dark brown, nearly black center. Black-eyed susans were for Dad. As the flowers die back in the fall, gold finches eat the seeds as we watch from the porch.

Orange daylilies dug up from the side of the road filled the second tier. Orange day lilies were a nod to Keith's and my wedding. They bloomed early the year we were married and provided a natural back-drop to the festivities. Besides, hummingbirds enjoyed their trumpet-shaped flowers. I also had purple irises with their yellow caterpillar like beard. The grass like foliage of deep purple Siberian irises moves gently in the wind. These were for Momma, to be truthful, there are few flowers that don't spark some memory of Momma because we planted so many together.

the third and lowest tier held coreopsis, it's tiny yellow flowers with a yellow center blossomed on mounds of delicate green leaves. Inter-spersed among the coreopsis were coral bells. Their thin spires, lined with red bell-shaped flowers, rose from a mound of dark green leaves.

I filled the shaded section of the lowest tier with hostas that came from Momma's flower beds. Hostas are one of the few plants I enjoy as much for their foliage as their blossoms. Their green leaves are often variegated with white or yellow. The shades of green can run from a deep blue green to pale, almost lime green. Hosta's bell-shaped blossoms of pale blue or white also form along a tall spire.

The overall effect was more like an English cottage garden. In an English cottage garden, plants appear to be chosen and placed willy-nilly throughout the bed, but the gardener works out where to put each plant. In the end, they all came together for a pleasing visual. I've never been drawn to regimented formal gardens.

Over Easter, we took a trip to Virginia to visit Momma. It was so good to see her. Although she tried to hide it, I could tell that her respiratory issues were getting worse. Of course, her spring was well ahead of ours. I took back iris rhizomes, sedum, hens and chicks, and a couple of different hostas. The sedum really helped soften the slate I used for terracing.

Once school was out, we took a trip to Johns Island to visit my Uncle Butch and stopped along the way to see my Aunt Judy. Retired from the mill, she now made floral arrangements for weddings and other events. She took to the kids right away and shot basketball with them. I had forgotten that she played softball while in school. She followed us to Johns Island a couple of days later.

Although Kenny and Keith had traveled to Hawaii so Kenny could play baseball as part of the Young Ambassadors program, Sarah had never seen the beach. We slathered her in sunscreen to keep her from getting sunburned. We boiled and ate shrimp in the backyard. Butch and Judy took us around Charleston. The kids got to see the Battery where I played as a child. Butch showed us places he and Grandpa had built. We took a drive over to the Isle of Palms, where I lived for a while when Terry was a baby. There was so much new construction. Of course, the house I lived in was gone. No longer the peaceful middle class island. It had become just another resort area.

I felt rested and connected to my family and myself. After talking things over with Keith, I resolved I would find work closer to home. Even though I loved being a director of nursing, the three hours travel every day was too much.

26

Time Folding

In 2002, I took a day supervisor position at a skilled nursing facility in Wellsboro. My shift started at 630 every morning and was supposed to end at 230 in the afternoon. I supervised the care of 150 residents while I was on duty. About 60 of them were receiving skilled services from either the therapy department or nursing. There were two unit managers, but their primary functions were care planning and family meetings. At least the facility was only 30 minutes away. The pay wasn't great, but I got a shift differential and overtime when I had to stay over at a change of shift. This happened a lot. At least, I didn't take work home with me.

Things seemed better, and then they turned into a blur. I worked more hours than I can remember. My 630 to 230 shifts often lasted until six in the evening as I processed orders I had received during the day. We always needed more money for something, so I didn't complain. An opportunity for Kenny or Sarah. Or something for the house, which we were still trying to improve enough so it would qualify for a VA loan. I was back to being unable to sleep. Often, I would be almost asleep and then I would stare at the doctor's list on my closed eyelids. *Is everything checked off? Did I miss anything?* Sleep deprivation distorts everything. There were so many good things that happened while we lived there. But it's hard for me to parse it out in true chronological order.

Keith supplemented our income working basketball camps, which often took him away. Keith's family stopped coming up as often after Dad died. I got down to Virginia to see Momma twice. She came up from Virginia to celebrate Thanksgiving in 2002. She helped me work on my Broken Dishes quilt. I had chosen the colors to go with the dishes I used and several that I kept on display.

Once they were in junior high school, both kids played for the school teams and continued to do so through high school. Kenny played football for a season and Sarah played a season of soccer. In the summer, there were basketball camps. The only time Keith and I both weren't both at a game was when the kids had a game on the same day.

We went back to Nokesville for Jimmy's wedding. Momma helped me prepare sandwich platters and tiny chocolate pies for the simple rehearsal dinner requested by the couple. Despite her breathing problems, Momma attended the wedding.

While Kenny and Sarah were in high school, Keith started working for a tree company in Baltimore. He stayed with his sister and came home most weekends. This wasn't our favorite choice, but it needed to be done. At least by this time, Kenny was driving. And while it was good that he could do some of the driving to practices. I worried about his impetuous nature.

Momma decided that she wanted to move to Texas and be near her youngest grandchildren. I tried to talk her into moving to Pennsylvania, but she felt the weather and pollen from the trees would be too much for her. In the end, I went to Virginia on a couple of weekends to help her pack. Keith brought the truck on the last trip, so we could take the things we had in the garage up to the cabin. With the help of my Aunt BJ and Martin, Momma moved into a two-bedroom house in Paris, Texas. She was catty-corner across the street from my brother.

Momma and I wrote letters and talked on the phone. Texas so far away. I missed her terribly. In the fall, I got a call from my aunt. Momma wasn't doing well. I flew to Texas for a visit. I helped her organize the house. She had gotten a chihuahua, Tiger. He barked at me when I first came in. Tiger didn't really like me much. He was probably just jealous and defensive. Mostly, I tried to catch her up on things with the kids. She had sold her car, so she didn't get out much. We planned a trip in the spring so I could help her get her front yard in shape.

Not long after, we made the trip to Waukegan for David's wedding. Tammie's family was gracious and planned meals for everyone living out of town. It was good to see David. I was sorry that Momma couldn't be there. I sent her lots of pictures.

As planned, Sarah and I made a road trip to Texas as soon as school was out. Kenny had basketball camps, so he stayed home. On the way, we picked up Terry and Ben in Virginia. Ben navigated using a road atlas while Terry and Sarah sat in the back. We made an overnight stop in Tennessee, but mostly we drove. Listening and singing along to Lynyrd Skynyrd's "Home Alabama" and "Simple Man" to stay awake.

Finally, we made it to Texas. The flattest, scrubbiest land I have ever seen not connected to a beach. I knew Momma used oxygen all the time, but now she's using a walker. She had old brick piled up to border the flower beds and make a small area for a bench in the front yard. Two planting beds were to go along the front of the house and another along the edge of the driveway. She also had peat moss to amend the soil.

We started out with shovels. After Martin borrowed a tiller, getting the soil ready went much faster. Once we had the soil amended, Momma and I went to the nursery to pick out her plants. Of course, there were hostas, irises, snapdragons, and holly trees. Momma liked holly trees with berries. We also used sweet potato vine as a ground cover. By dinner, we had the holly trees planted.

The next two days were a flurry of planting and mulching. Sarah and Terry planted right along with me. Benny was working on the small seating area. It was hot. Momma, unable physically to work with us, kept watch from the shade and frequently reminded us to take a break.

"Sherry, you're not a construction worker. It's 101 out here. Get over in the shade, take a break, and drink some water."

"Okay, Momma. We're coming. Gotta water this plant in."

We all sat for a bit. Sarah told Momma about school and her friends in Pennsylvania. We laughed as we made jokes about doing an HGTV yard makeover and having a big reveal tomorrow afternoon. Their laughter was wonderful to hear. Momma got tired and went inside. We went back to planting. In the evening, I worked on the quilt I was making for my grandson, who was due in August. Momma helped me with the final layout of the blocks. I'm not sure who was more excited, me at having a grandchild or Momma at being a great grandmother.

We finished up in the yard late morning just before lunch. We took a ton of pictures, which I promised to send to Momma. At home, I even put them together in an album. Later that afternoon, a friend of my brother took family pictures. Those were the last ones ever taken of us as a family.

The following August, our first grandson was born. We all made another trip to Waukegan to welcome him and present him with the quilt I made for him. Again, we stayed with Tammie's family. As excited as I was to be a grandmother, I was unprepared for the way he wrapped himself around my heart. Too soon, we had to return to Pennsylvania.

I had always known I wanted to be a grandmother. No rush. I was happy to wait until the couples decided they were ready. Never in my wildest dreams did I expect to feel a similar bond as when I held each of my children for the first time. There are no words to describe it. It's simply amazing.

27

Texas Again

We had gone to Baltimore to visit Keith's sister, Claudia. While there, we did some early Christmas shopping. As we purchased framed photos of Cal Ripken for the boys, I saw an artist's rendition of Fenway Park as they won the 2004 World Series. Keith was such a big Red Sox fan. I knew it would be the perfect Christmas gift for him. I arranged for his sister to purchase it for me and mail it to the cabin.

Once we were back home, Keith started working on a propane central heating system. Funny thing though, while setting in some of the ductwork, Keith cut into his Christmas gift without knowing it. I had hidden it behind a cedar chest and up against a wall, determined to keep it a secret. Unable to replace it, we gave it to him, anyway. He felt so terrible, but disguised the cut since it was in the stands. It was not noticeable unless you looked closely. He loved it anyway. Years later, Kenny and April gave him a duplicate.

In early November, I got a call from my brother in Texas. Momma wasn't doing well and was needing more help. Could I see if I could work something out? Another flight out of Newark, NJ. If you weren't in a negative state of mind before, the drive into Newark would do it.

Thirty years later, scars of summer riots remained. It was clear the city had done some rebuilding and the downtown area definitely showed the effects of some revitalization. But just a few blocks away, weeds filled vacant lots next to boarded-up buildings. As we drove past, most of the homes we saw were neat and well kept, despite the empty lots where homes or businesses would have stood.

Momma now has a motorized wheelchair. She had fallen in the bathroom and deep bruises in various shades of purple, red, and yellow covered her face and forearms. During the warmest part of the day, we would take Tiger for a walk as she motored slowly along in her wheelchair. She introduced me to some of her neighbors as we made the rounds.

Back at the house, I read aloud to her as she sat in her recliner. "I just want to hear your voice," she said. Often, she drifted off to sleep. Prednisone taken to relieve her asthma was driving her weight up. Momma had been slender most of her life and she was very conscious of her weight gain. Besides, cooking and eating drained her energy reserves. It was hard to get her to eat a nutritious meal even when I cooked it.

While I was there with the help of her doctor, I arranged for a home health aide to come in three days a week. He also signed off on my FMLA paperwork. I collaborated with the home health nurse as she set up Momma's weekly pill box. Momma was uncomfortable with the idea of someone giving her a shower.

"I don't mind them doing the light housekeeping and laundry. But I don't want them giving me a shower. I don't like people seeing me or touching me that aren't family," Momma told me after the nurse left.

"We're afraid of your falling again. Let's go in the bathroom and see if we can work out a way to get you safely in the shower so you can bathe yourself. You already have the shower chair."

Sally Rand may have been famous for her fan dance, but Momma and I developed a robe/towel dance that allowed her to maintain her privacy and dignity while an aide could ensure her safety. Momma would undress and get into her robe while sitting on the side of her bed. Her aide would come in to see her safely in the shower. Once in the shower, Momma would remove her robe and hand it to her aide. The aide waited outside the shower curtain while Momma bathed. When Momma was through, the aide handed Momma her towel. Momma dried off and put on her robe behind the shower curtain. The aide helped her step out of the tub.

After a couple of dry runs on our own, I wrote out the steps and trained her aide when she came in the first time. We left a copy in her bathroom closet. The home health nurse added to Momma's care plan.

Momma made a point of showing her appreciation. "You're always so patient. You never complained. Nobody understands what you've done over the years. All the appointments, hospital visits, helping me in the house and yard. But I do."

"Aw, Momma. It's what children should do. Help their parents when they need it. You took care of all of us."

"You and Keith are great parents. You've raised some good kids. I'm proud of you."

"Thanks Momma." Never able to accept compliments well, I went to get dinner ready. Momma fell asleep again, but not before she made me promise to take Tiger home with me if she was away from home for a long time. Neither of us wanted to talk about the possibility of her dying.

After dinner, I was packing to leave in the morning. Momma had me gather up some old dressmaker shears and a salesman's model for a Singer sewing machine. The largest pair of scissors had five-inch blades and looked like a prop for a horror movie.

"Momma, TSA's going to check my bags. They might take these scissors away from me."

"Just put them in between your clothes. It will be okay."

Early the next morning, I left for my flight out of Dallas. I cried most of the fight. I was afraid this would be the last time I saw Momma alive.

28

Quilted Northern

I had been working as an MDS coordinator at the same facility for a couple of years now. The pace was still stressful, but there were no lists on my ceiling at night. When I returned to work, the renovations for my new office were complete. I no longer had a shared space with the other MDS coordinator. There was just enough room for a desk, a file cabinet, and a visitor's chair. At least it had a window. I moved files and got settled in.

At home, we started up the basketball season. Keith was now refereeing basketball games. The merry-go-round of who had a game today resumed. Keith's siblings made it to a few games. Thanksgiving and Christmas came and went. I talked with Momma on the phone. Sent her cards and letters with pictures of the kids.

In January, the long dreaded phone call came. Momma was in the hospital again. She had fallen. Momma was also having a flareup of her COPD and asthma. She hadn't been able to maintain her oxygen levels, even with her home oxygen. After giving them time to get her settled, I called the hospital. Momma was drowsy, unable to communicate clearly. The hospital nurses couldn't add much more to what my brother had told me.

I started looking into having Momma transferred to the assisted living facility connected to the facility where I worked. Since she was a family member of an employee, there would be a discount on the monthly fee. I could provide things like help with bathing and laundry. These add-ons always drove up the price. It would be expensive, but with all the family's help, it would be manageable. They could sell or rent the house in Texas to give her more income.

All that planning didn't matter. The doctor intubated her and hoped to get her off the ventilator in a few days. Her oxygen saturation kept dropping each time the doctors tried to remove the breathing tube. She was being transferred to a long-term hospital or LTAC.

After calling Jimmy and David to figure out how they would get to Texas. Keith, Kenny, Sarah, and I started planning our trip. We would pick Jimmy up in Virginia. Our only stops were for food and bathroom breaks. Twenty-three hours straight, we drove. David flew into Dallas from Chicago.

All the family was there. Ben and Terry, my aunts and uncle. At first, Momma was alert and smiling. She recognized everyone and tried to communicate with us. Her left hand had an IV, so she had trouble trying to write. Bruises from failed attempts to gain IV access covered her right hand. At her request, we took turns reading to her. Momma smiled as Kenny and Sarah told her about school and basketball. She pantomimed questions about her great grandson.

The next day, Momma began fighting her breathing tube. Quite a normal reaction, but that meant the doctor increased her sedation. I encouraged everyone to talk to or read to her as I did even though she couldn't talk. She would squeeze our hand to let us know she heard us. There were so many of us that the hospital set up a lounge area in a room on a closed wing so that we wouldn't take over the waiting room or disturb anyone on the unit. By some fluke, Keith, the kids, and I had red or black coats. We must have been a sight going up the hallways. Keith and our tall boys surrounding Sarah and me protectively.

We visited in shifts. Some would go to back to Momma's so they could sleep in an actual bed and bring back food for those at the hospital. We got to know all the nurses and her doctor. Momma no longer needed antibiotics, but they still couldn't ween her from the breathing tube. She was being fed through a tube.

I tried to talk to Aunt BJ about getting Momma into palliative care, but she didn't think this was the time. She saw the change as "giving up". Since she and I were both Momma's medical power of attorney, we needed to agree.

With no definitive prognosis, the family started drifting back to their homes. I was thankful all my children had seen her alert. Momma played such a large role in their lives. My Aunt BJ would stay longer as she had her own business. Her daughter would spell her when BJ needed to go back to Virginia. We took Tiger with us. Poor little dog never adjusted to the cold or life away from Momma.

Life in Pennsylvania returned to familiar routines. Work, basketball games and dinners with family. I spoke with my aunt, brother, or Momma's nurses every day. But there was no change until the end of February. My cousin called to say the nurses were trying to draw blood because she needed a blood transfusion, but Momma kept crying and pulling her arm away.

I called the hospital. The nurse couldn't tell me why they were doing transfusions. Only that Momma's hemoglobin was low. *Did she have internal bleeding? Is her body decreasing the number of red bloods it made?* She couldn't give me an answer. As one of Momma's medical power of attorneys, I had them stop the blood draws and hold off on the transfusion.

After talking with Martin, Terry, and Benny, I started the drive to Texas. I would pick up Terry and Benny in Virginia along with my Aunt Judy and Aunt Shirley. It upset Kenny and Sarah that I wouldn't take them with me.

"I want to go with you to see Grandmother." Kenny complained.

"Me too," Sarah chimed in.

"Not this time. Grandmother's really sick. She won't know you're there."

Kenny was in his senior year of high school. College scouts were coming to his basketball games. Neither one of them needed to be out of school. Besides, I was going down to get her started on palliative care. I wanted the kids to remember her when she was smiling and trying to communicate with us. And to remember all the wonderful times they had with her. While I knew her death wouldn't be immediate, I didn't think she would be with us long once the doctor removed her breathing tube. I'd explained this process to many families, but chickened out telling my children.

Judy shared the driving, so we drove straight to Texas. After a brief stop at Momma's house, we went to the hospital. The doctor had Momma deeply sedated so she wouldn't fight the ventilator. She didn't respond to our voices or touch. Her only responses were to cry out in pain when the nurses repositioned her. All the family agreed it was time to let Momma go. There was a family meeting with her doctor. BJ and I, as her medical powers of attorney, expressed the family's opinion that this wasn't what Momma would call life and asked for the breathing tube to be removed. He agreed and scheduled it for the next day.

Many times, people think once you remove the things keeping a loved one alive, death occurs immediately. In reality, it takes time, and it's hard to predetermine how long that will be. Momma's breathing tube was out. The feeding tube was out. Her IV fluids had been stopped. The nurses removed the equipment from her room and brought in a courtesy cart, so no one had to leave Momma to get coffee or a snack.

We sat by her bedside, rotating positions to be close to her. Her restlessness subsided as I held her hand and whispered. "It's okay, Momma. All your babies have grown up and are doing well. It's okay to rest now. You don't have to fight anymore. I love you." The nurses came in quietly to administer the morphine and provide other care to keep Momma comfortable.

Finally, long after the sandwiches on the cart had grown stale, Momma's breathing became more difficult. She began picking at the bedcovers and tossing her head from side to side. I went to the nurses' station and requested Momma's nurse to give the next dose of morphine. A few minutes later, the nurse came into the room with the morphine and a syringe.

"You know, this could seriously decrease her respiratory rate."

Her pulse oximeter was showing about eighteen respirations a minute. Momma was panting, and she still tossed her head from side to side on the pillow.

I glanced at my aunt, willing her to agree with me. She nodded yes. "Go ahead. Carolyn's having such a hard time."

I held Momma's hand as the nurse administered the medication and resumed my whispers of love. The rest of the family gathered close around the bedside. Within a few minutes, Momma closed her eyes for the last time. Peacefully.

Except for the few minutes it took the nurses to do postmortem care, we stayed at her bedside until the funeral home came to pick her up. Somehow, we got back to Momma's house. I called home to let Keith and the kids know.

Uncle Butch, the man I'd only seen drink an occasional beer, pulled a bottle of peach schnapps from his suitcase. After we each took a couple of shots, I curled up in Momma's recliner with a blanket. Tomorrow, I would have to follow the driver from the funeral home to the crematorium. Momma made us promise we would see her cremated to be sure it happened. She watched a show where an unscrupulous funeral home dumped the bodies in the woods after collecting the fees. We were to be sure her body went into the crematorium. But tonight, I slept dreaming of Momma's smiling face.

My aunts and uncle left the day after the funeral. Judy and Shirley flew back with Uncle Butch. They would spread her ashes at my grandma's graveside in Charleston before returning home.

There wasn't much to do with wrapping up Momma's affairs. She had a life insurance policy that took care of her funeral expenses. Her legacy was love and the things she taught us. My siblings and I took a few days sorting out Momma's things, deciding what to keep or donate.

I spent most of this time in a fog. I was relieved that Momma was no longer struggling, but I was angry. I was sad. Since no one would leave me alone, I couldn't just cry.

Finally, we left Texas, and I made it back home after dropping Ben and Terry in Virginia. The whirlwind of our lives there picked me up and kept me going. I longed for spring, even though it meant Kenny's graduation from high school would come soon.

I was growing restless and bored with my job. The facility's renovations put everyone in small offices, causing more isolation. It was harder to connect to the staff and residents. There was no promotion in sight. My boss had been doing her job for years and would never leave until she retired. I was tired of being harassed into taking shifts as a supervisor or as a charge nurse because the facility couldn't hire enough nurses to cover everything. Thinking I might become an administrator, I enrolled in an online health care administration program. Maybe then I could have a positive impact on nurses' working conditions and the care of residents in a facility.

Sarah was having trouble with a molar, and Keith took her into the dentist. Since she had an abscess, the dentist prescribed antibiotics and pain medication. She was to return in a week. Because of the snow, Keith stayed home with her, and I went in to work. About 2 in the afternoon, Keith calls me. He's concerned because her face was so swollen. I hurry home. My sweet girl's oval face has swollen so much she now has a jawline to rival Jay Leno. We bundle her up and take her to the emergency room.

The snow falls so thickly we can hardly see as Keith lets Sarah and me out by the door while he parks the car. Nurses quickly get us into a treatment room. Sarah's crying with huge tears running down her face as she tries not to yell out as the staff assess her mouth. It's determined that an oral surgeon needs to see Sarah. It's Friday, our dentist has gone away for the weekend. Wellsboro is a small town; there's not another oral surgeon.

During the hours we were in the emergency room, the snow turned into a blizzard. The nearest oral surgeons are over an hour away. Our family doctor, Keith and I decide it would be better to admit Sarah to the hospital here overnight for observation and give her IV fluids. With IV access, the nurses could manage her pain better than I could at home with oral medication. In the morning, she could be transported by ambulance to the Children's Hospital in Danville.

With the heavy snow, it was late afternoon when we arrived in Danville. I had carried copies of Sarah's medical record from the hospital and was able to hand them over when the hospitalist seemed confused by our presence. We would see the oral surgeon in the morning. Janet Weiss Children's Hospital was perfect for us. The nurses were fantastic. They allowed me to help Sarah as I was able. There was plenty of room for me to be with her without crowding the staff.

Being part of a large teaching hospital meant there would be medical students with the hospitalist assigned, since the oral surgeon couldn't follow Sarah medically. Most of the time, this worked well for us. However, once the oral surgeon pulled her tooth, there was a bit of back and forth about criteria for Sarah's discharge. Sarah and I were becoming discouraged. Our surgeon put his foot down and gave the clear direction I was looking for. We convinced the Sarah that managing her pain meant using her PCA pump and not letting her pain level get out of control. Things progressed well. She soon weaned herself off the IV medications and we went home.

It was a surreal time for me. All the emotions that go with having a child in the hospital, even when you know their illness is not as serious as other children on the unit, threatened to overwhelm me. The hospital was very nice. They sent a tray for me at mealtimes. There was a small laundry room for parents, a lounge area, and vending machines. Mostly, I watched movies with Sarah. Keith came to visit Sarah but needed to work. So, while Sarah slept, I was again wandering a hospital in a town I didn't know. I knew Sarah would be fine, but this was too soon after Momma's death. All the water was frozen and my personal cloud was dark.

29

The Nest Empties

Spring finally came. The county government forced the hotel to put in a special grease disposal unit and lock up their trash dumpster to keep the bear from foraging in them. Apparently, eating human food waste will leave the bear prone to a variety of diseases. While this policy offered some benefits for the bear, it meant the bear began joining deer in their trek across the flat with more frequency.

One night, crashing trash cans sent Champ racing out of his dog door. As the tone of his barking changed, Keith went out to investigate. Champ had treed a bear cub right next to the porch landing. The small tree swayed under the bear's weight and looked as if it would break as it bent nearly to the ground. Eventually, the bear dropped and ran up a larger tree, but Champ and eventually Tiger kept running in an arc around the tree and barking. Finally, Keith got the dogs inside and, from the safety of the porch, we watched the bear drop down and lumber off.

In June, Kenny graduated. Although very intelligent, Kenny was more invested in basketball than studying. He set the record for points scored at his high school. We had a huge celebration for Kenny on the flat—barbeque with all the family and his friends. He planned to go to Greensboro College in North Carolina, where he would play basketball. We spent the summer purchasing things for his dorm room.

That September, I took him to Greensboro. We stopped in Franklin, Virginia, to see Jimmy. Kenny was so excited and kept trying to reassure me he would be fine. His dorm mates were already there. All of them were basketball players and they wanted to get to know each other. They helped get his stuff into the room and I headed on back to Pennsylvania. I was happy he could live this part of his dream. I managed not to cry as Kenny walked me to the car. A block away in a parking lot, I cried like a baby.

Kenny didn't come home for Thanksgiving because of basketball commitments. Jimmy was in Virginia for Thanksgiving. Keith, Sarah, and I drove to Waukegan to see David and his family. We had Thanksgiving dinner with Tammie's family. Strange not to have them all with me.

Life was a little less hectic with only one student athlete. Keith and I continued going to all her games. Sarah was always an excellent student. She continued playing softball and basketball for the high school. Her senior year, she won several scholarships and the Future Young Leaders award for the county. As a catcher, she set the school's record for getting people out as they tried to get to second base. She continued working.

After her graduation, we held another celebration on the flat. Family and friends were all there. We rented cabins from a neighbor for all the out-of-town guests. After visiting several schools, Sarah decided Mary Baldwin in Virginia was the school for her. We spent the rest of the summer working, helping me in the yard and gathering things for her dorm room.

At the end of August, I drove her to Mary Baldwin. There were a lot of young women to help us get things to her third-floor dorm room. We set up her cappuccino machine and other things. We made a trip to Walmart to pick up curtains and some food. She was so excited to start the next phase of her life. It was wonderful to see. Again, once away from the school, I cried.

30

Last Winter

Keith and I went through the days. Thanksgiving rolled around again. Jimmy, Sarah, and Kenny made it home. They breathed life into the cabin while they were there. We went to Waukegan to see David. I cooked Thanksgiving dinner. Too soon we all returned to our regular lives.

The winter was brutal. Snow covered everything. Open areas sparkled with frozen snow, but anything near the road was grimy and dark gray from cinders spread on the road for traction. The lake I passed on the way to work had frozen over and was dotted with tents put up by ice fishermen. Subzero temperatures for days, without an end in sight. Keith was away from home working on storm damage. I detested it. One evening, while talking with Keith on the phone, I told him I wanted to look for work in Virginia. The cabin wasn't anything without family here. He agreed. I turned in my thirty-day notice at work and started sending out resumes online. I began packing.

I decorated for Christmas, even though for the first time, my heart wasn't in it. But Sarah and Kenny would be home, and it needed to be right for them. Keith made it home on Christmas Eve. All too soon, I had to take Sarah and Kenny back to school. Keith went back to work.

I made a trip to Roanoke for an interview but didn't like the facility. Sarah and I watched Barack Obama's acceptance speech on television. There was so much hope.

On the way back to Pennsylvania, I talked on the phone with David. He mentioned seeing a news segment about nurse shortages in North Carolina. I still held my Virginia nursing license and North Carolina was one of the compact states. I broadened my search. After a few telephone interviews with recruiters and human resources personnel, I set up in-person interviews. Keith and I decided I would fly to Greensboro since my car wasn't the most reliable.

Kenny and a friend picked me up at the airport in Greensboro, where he and Jimmy had an apartment. I would stay with them for a couple of days and borrow a car to go to my interviews. I interviewed at a facility outside of Charlotte but still had interviews in Statesville and Chapel Hill. In the end I chose Chapel Hill. They didn't quibble about my salary requirements and offered excellent an excellent sign-on bonus that would help with moving expenses. Besides, Kenny and Jimmy were in Greensboro, and it wasn't too far from Mary Baldwin.

Thinking of our time in Pennsylvania always brings up conflicting emotions for me. It was beautiful. It was peaceful. I loved gardening there. The soil was amazing. We could give the kids more freedom to roam than we ever could have done in Marshall. I made a few good friends. There was a natural swimming hole within walking distance of the back door. Sarah made a lifelong friend. I worked with wonderful nurses and doctors. We had a lot of good times there.

But it was more insular than anywhere I've ever lived. I'm sure I contributed to some of the feeling of isolation and alienation. We struggled so hard, and I was too proud to let anyone know about the financial difficulties we faced. Forget talking about depression. For healthcare professionals, there's still a serious stigma that stops us from talking about our mental health issues. In the end, summers were short. Winter was cold. It was dark.

31

Starting Over--Again

The last week of December 2008, I said goodbye to the snow covered ground of Pennsylvania. I stopped to see Sarah in Staunton and stayed overnight in a hotel before heading on to Greensboro. At first, I would stay with Jimmy and Kenny in their apartment. Keith would stay at the cabin until I found us a place to live. He was making good money working storm damage.

The daily trip to Chapel Hill was an hour each way when traffic was moving. On the way home, traffic slowed to a crawl as US 40 narrowed from four lanes to two. Without a GPS, I had a hard time learning my way around Greensboro. Who am I kidding? I still get lost in Greensboro, even with a GPS.

By mid-January, I started looking for houses. I wanted to be closer to work. Eventually, I focused on Burlington. Its location between Chapel Hill and Greensboro was ideal should I later decide to change jobs. Besides, I liked the feeling I got while traveling around town. It was large enough to have the amenities I wanted and yet small enough to appeal to the small-town girl in me.

Kenny and I drove out to see a house in Burlington. Although it was noisy because of its proximity to Interstate 40, it had a lot of room. Two bedrooms, eat-in kitchen, dining room, living room upstairs with another bedroom, family room, laundry room and bathroom downstairs. There would be enough room when everyone came to visit.

Besides the noise, it was strange getting used to the glow of city lights above trees. One night coming in after covering an evening shift, I looked up at the sky and was amazed by how few stars were visible. Definitely an "oh duh" moment. Blackwell didn't have streetlights, so when the sky was clear, the stars truly shone like diamonds. Here, even the brightest were like pinpoints.

In the end, Kenny moved back in with us. Jimmy and a friend would keep the apartment in Greensboro. It took until June for Keith to get everything down from Pennsylvania and finish closing up the cabin. Eventually, all the kids would come back, at different times, to live with us in that house.

At first, Keith looked for work with a tree company. Everyone here thought a climber in their 50s was too old. Eventually, he made a few connections and started his own business. It grew to include landscaping, handyman type home repairs and mowing construction sites in developments.

Trying to stay connected to the young adults my children had become, we started a family recreational pool team. I was out of my element. Except for my earlier years in the Navy, I had never been involved in the bar scene. It was actually quite fun because we did it together. We made it to the league playoffs a few times and even took third place once.

I shifted from working as an MDS coordinator back to being a director of nursing (DON). My niche was working to get troubled facilities back up to par. Back to horrific hours and being on call all the time. It was rewarding to realize that you helped make changes that affected others' lives.

It was also eye opening. I met a black nurse who was among the first to work at UNC Hospital when it desegregated. Other black women told me about growing up in Chapel Hill and how they had to be careful where they went to avoid unwanted attention or outright discrimination. Still, they felt privileged having grown up as daughters of professionals in Chapel Hill.

Kenny enlisted in the Army. Playing basketball in college was not what he thought it would be. Of course, there was also the cost of attending a four-year college. Even though I had done service in the Navy and Keith in the Army, it's another thing when your son tells you he's going to do this. We had troops in Afghanistan and were sending more. I applauded his decision to take control of his life, but my mother's heart was terrified for him.

Jimmy completed his bachelor's degree in 2011. Keith was working out of town. Sarah and I attended his graduation. I was and continue to be so proud of him.

David moved in with us about this time. Keith rented a trailer to get him moved down from Illinois. While they weren't all living with us, for the first time in many years, all my children were in the same state.

In March, the facility I worked in just finished a nearly perfect CMS survey and was removed from the special focus list. This involved 18 months of grueling work to ensure the facility was adhering to CMS regulations and any plans of correction that were put in place. After enduring CMS surveys every six months, the facility's corporate owners announced we were closing. We went from excitedly planning staff celebrations to dumbfounded confusion in the space of 24 hours.

We needed to find new homes for the 135 people living in the facility. The residents in the dementia unit would be the first to be transferred. As more people were transferred, we merged the two remaining units to simplify staffing. Staff layoffs started. Sister facilities began picking up equipment. By June, we found facilities for all residents. Walking through the building was a surreal experience. The memory of all the hard work, the people who had worked and lived here was so strong I felt they might appear as spirits in the quiet hallways. After a last walk through with a corporate representative, the administrator and I turned in our keys.

I took a DON position in a Greensboro facility owned by the same corporation. The same problems plagued this facility as the one in Chapel Hill: staffing shortages, low admission rates, and a lot of complaints. Newly renovated, the facility looked good.

Unlike the Chapel Hill facility, I didn't have a full complement of administrative nurses or supervisors. There was very little cushion between me and the frequent nursing call outs. Adding the need for in-services and audits on all three shifts, I began a year and a half of literally coming home to sleep for four hours and then going back to work. If I made it home for an evening, my phone was always ringing with a nurse reporting an incident or problem and I had to walk them through the initial part of an investigation. It wasn't that the nurse was necessarily incompetent. It was policy. Keith stopped asking when I would come home from work. I did not know. I called when I was on my way home.

Struggling with low admission rates led to our administrator to work out an agreement to accept some hospital patients who needed skilled nursing care but didn't have insurance. The hospital would start the Medicaid application process. Then the facility would have a payor source to bill once the patient's Medicaid was approved. This led to some atypical admissions: people younger than the general population and people with mental health or substance use problems. It was difficult to meet all their needs. Our activities were geared toward people in their 60s and older, the usual population for SNFs.

A young woman, Elise, in her late twenties, was a perfect example of the problems that often occurred with these types of admissions. Elise came to us with a large wound on her upper arm just above her elbow. She had been using krokodil and the resulting lesions became infected. Our social worker tried working with her regarding her substance use disorder and to develop ways to keep her engaged while in the facility since she always stated, "there's nothing to do here "and wanted to go out. Leaving the facility could be problematic for a couple of reasons. The resident would miss treatments and delay healing. From a billing point of view, if the resident could leave frequently, they could be treated at home and didn't need to be in a SNF.

Elise had a male friend who visited periodically. After being in the facility for about a week, Elise reported her grandmother had died and received permission to go to the funeral. She left with the male friend who had been visiting.

Sitting at the nurses station while doing chart reviews, I looked up to see a bright red dot on the hallway floor. Getting up and going down the hall, I realize the dot is blood and there is a trail leading to a room. I call for housekeeping and the crash cart as I follow the trail.

My team of nurses and the nurse practitioner who was rounding immediately followed me into Elise's room. Elise was barely conscious, lying face down on her bed. Apparently, her friend snuck her back in and left her and his bloody jacket on the bed. Blood soaked towels, obviously not ones used by the SNF, wrapped around her left arm. As we worked frantically, the paramedics were called. One nurse got IV access in her right arm and started fluids as I began slowly unwrapping the towels. Blood shot up from the wound. An arterial bleed. After applying a tourniquet, we removed the towels and redressed the wound with a pressure bandage.

The paramedics arrived and took Elise to the hospital. Her vitals were still erratic as they loaded her on the ambulance. Putting her linens in biohazard bags, I realized I had a large amount of blood on my uniform, probably from when I helped reposition Elise. Driving home to change, I prayed she was not HIV positive. After showering and changing uniforms, I made the 35 minute drive back to work to conclude the audit I had been conducting. When questioning the receptionist later, she told me Elise's friend had carried her into the building and declined a wheelchair, saying he didn't want to wake her.

We later found out Elise survived and eventually went to another facility. She was not HIV positive. It troubled me her companion just left her bleeding on the bed without telling us she was in trouble. Elise was a human being, not a bit of flotsam to be tossed aside once she was no longer useful.

Keith and I finally made it away for a three-day weekend to the beach. When I returned, my administrator had rewritten my nursing schedule for the next month with nothing but 12-hour shifts and not all the shifts were covered. She made it clear that changing the schedule would cost me my job. Many people in healthcare, including some nurses, feel 12-hour shifts are the answer to nursing shortages. It might look good on paper but, when a call off occurs it is harder to fill a shift. Getting someone to pick up part of an eight-hour shift means they'll be working 12 hours. Often a nurse will stay for an extra four hours or come in four hours early. If it's a 12-hour shift, then you're looking at working for 16 hours. Finally, as the manager, you must consider how long they'll be off before they're working again. The stuff of nightmares.

All of this eventually made me question whether or not I would continue with my nursing career. It wouldn't have been so bad but, there was no appreciation, no approval for the small things I wanted to do to raise morale in the nursing department. Instead of giving in-services about becoming better nurses, I spent my time writing plans of correction and in-servicing staff on how to avoid a deficiency during state inspections. Then there were the audits to ensure nurses maintained the standard. And then auditing the auditors. A giant whirlpool sucked me deeper into the ocean and away from the sun. My blood pressure was again causing concern. Eventually, I resigned.

This was the first time I considered leaving the nursing profession. I was angry and frustrated with a system which discounted nurses' needs or often simply ignored them. Many administrators and corporate personal act as if nurses are disposable. I've had administrators say, "nurses are a dime a dozen".

Without consulting nurses, non-nurses make decisions regarding patient care and the processes by which nurses deliver care. This occurs in hospitals and SNFs but has been historically worse in SNF's. Nurses then must provide care to an ever-increasing number of patients. All this leads to poorer patient outcomes, no matter how skilled or dedicated the nurse is.

32

Life's About Changes

Keith and I, along with David, moved to a quieter neighborhood in Burlington. For a short period, I did a few contract jobs. I wasn't ready to jump back into a facility and was not sure I would even continue working as a nurse. The hours for any administrative nursing position weren't conducive to maintaining a work life balance. As I already knew, those hours can snuff the passion out in a person.

I really enjoyed my last contract position, reviewing charts to capture billing. Most of the time, I worked from home with just a few site visits to upload records. Unfortunately, the hours were extremely variable, and the pay was less than I needed to stay financially solvent.

I finally connected increases in my depressive symptoms to periods where I felt I had little control of my situation. I don't have to control everyone else, just me. I learned to talk things through with Keith and arrive at a decision. The act of deciding, even if I couldn't act on the decision right away, was a major boon to my mental health.

Kenny returned from Afghanistan. He and April were getting married and wanted to have a barbeque in the backyard as their rehearsal dinner. Keith and I went into overdrive getting the flower beds and house ready. We planted bright red salvia to attract hummingbirds and purple cone plants. When a cone plant's blossom matures, it folds back and looks like a badminton birdie. Gold finches love their seeds. Of course, we planted tons of marigolds.

With Sarah's help, I made mounds of potato salad, gallons of baked beans, and appetizers galore. While we were at the wedding rehearsal, a dear friend took control of the grill for nearly endless racks of ribs covered in Keith's signature barbeque sauce. One of Keith's brothers and his sister made it for the wedding, as did my brother. It was such a wonderful gathering of family and friends. Shortly after the wedding, Kenny and April moved to Matthews.

Nursing still called to me. There are many ways to "be a nurse". I began looking at different areas of practice. Ultimately, I took a position as a nurse on an Assertive Community Treatment (ACT) team. An ACT team provides community mental health services to people with severe and persistent mental illness. Mental illness knows no socio-economic boundaries. However, for those without adequate resources, finding mental health care is extremely difficult. Our primary goal was to help these people avoid hospitalization, learn to manage their illness, and learn to navigate the health care system.

Working with marginalized people helped me grow as a person and as a professional. Even better, I had time to work with my clients and to understand why they were averse to certain aspects of healthcare. Maybe I could help them learn to access healthcare in a more beneficial way.

Stella was a good example of this. She had a diagnosis of schizophrenia and could be delusional sometimes. Stella had already learned to track her blood sugar four times a day and her blood pressure every morning. She recorded these in a composition notebook. Stella could answer most questions but usually took a roundabout way of getting to the meat of her problem. This made for some interesting home visits but didn't fit in with a doctor's busy schedule. My role when attending doctor's appointments was to be sure she understood the doctor's instructions and to keep her on track when answering questions.

While driving back from an appointment, she told me to "Find me another doctor. This man doesn't listen to me. I don't think he likes me."

"Why do you think he doesn't like you?"

"He's always fiddling with that computer. I don't think he hears me."

"I see. I don't like it when my doctor uses the computer while I'm there, but they don't give a doctor a lot of time to see patients."

"Oh."

"He's been doing a good job with your blood sugars and high blood pressure. Do you think you could give him another chance?"

"Well, he has been right about my medicine. Okay, nurse. I just wish he would listen."

"Okay, we'll work on a few things to help make this better for you. If they don't do the trick, I'll find you another doctor."

I started working with her to make a list of questions/symptoms for her doctor and how to get to the point quickly. Then we started role playing. We covered everything from making the appointment to checking out. For a while I continued to go with her to doctor's appointments, each time I would take a less active role. One of my proudest moments as a nurse came the day, I sat in the waiting room while she went to see her doctor alone. After checking out, Stella came up to me. Her face was lit up with the biggest smile. "I did it. He listened. I need to get a prescription filled. I don't have to come back for six months."

The SUV I purchased shortly after moving to North Carolina finally bit the dust. Although we were doing well, coming up with a down payment for a new car would be tough. About this time, Sarah and Jon wanted to sell his car. He was overseas and the car sat in the garage. Keith and I took over the payments.

Funny, learning how to help clients deal with anxiety taught me how to deal with my anxiety more effectively. For years, I tried to cope with my fears and anxiety by figuring out what the worst-case scenario could be in a situation. Then I would plan for whatever my anxious mind imagined. Not so bad but, then I would go over it repeatedly. It took me years to say, "*If it happens, I have a plan*" and let go rather than leaving the scenario on a constant feedback loop.

A similar thing happened regarding boundaries. Teaching my clients about personal boundaries, I realized I should take my own advice. For a while there were memes all over the internet about boundaries. My favorite is "no is a complete sentence". While it became cliché, it became my mantra when someone wanted to change on call days. A simple reminder that my "no" was enough.

A year after Kenny and April's wedding, Sarah and Jon got married. Another whirlwind of activity. Sarah's friend Catherine flew in to help with planning and other projects related to the wedding. Sarah, Keith, and I added to the flower beds. Another barbeque in the backyard for the wedding party and out-of-town guests. Jon was home a few days before heading back overseas.

Keith and I drove to Boston to see the Red Sox play. Riding the trains was an adventure. We played tourist, seeing as much of the town as possible on our brief trip. Boston is such a vibrant town. Except for quick trips to the beach, this was our first solo vacation in all our years of marriage. I love Boston Commons and the tiny public parks where the trains ran before, they went underground. A couple of years later, we repeated the trip with Sarah.

David was working in graphic design besides his regular job. He designed a sign for a business and several t-shirts. After a while, he moved into a townhouse. David had a daughter. Things were difficult for him here. Eventually, he moved back to Illinois with his biological dad.

Professionally, I became board certified in psychiatric mental health nursing. It involved a lot of independent study, continuing education, and another nursing licensure type test. My supervisor did send me to a lot of training, most of it free, but not all. The psychiatrist I worked with helped me sort out things I had difficulty understanding. I passed without difficulty. Becoming board certified made no difference in terms of job position or pay, but management always liked to point out my board certification during audits and surveys. Research shows that having board certified nurses on staff improves patient outcomes. Having been a nurse for many years, I didn't really expect much else from my employer. Being board certified wasn't a requisite for the position. I became board certified to improve my delivery of care and for a personal feeling of accomplishment.

I conducted a wellness class. It was very popular with our clients. Besides talking about nutrition and health maintenance, we role played various situations in the community---doctor visits, asking friends to go to a movie. Individually, I would take them grocery shopping or have cooking lessons in their home. I enjoyed it because the class allowed me to connect with the part of me that embraces public health nursing. To me, teaching someone ways to improve their health, physical or mental, is as important as giving them a pill.

While searching for class material, I came across mindfulness techniques to help break a worry anxiety loop that plagues many people. Mindfulness helps you stay in the moment because you focus on what is happening right now rather than on the track playing in your head. Several of my clients with schizophrenia found it helpful to distract them from their voices. Personally, I found mindfulness a great help with insomnia as well since my sleeplessness stemmed from not being able to "turn my brain off".

In my late fifties, I figured out I didn't *have* to fit in anywhere. My peers respected me professionally, my family loved me with all my quirks and foibles, and I was a decent human being. I stopped trying to be perfect or fit a particular mold. What a relief.

Sarah lived with Keith and me for a couple of years while Jon was working overseas. We grew even closer, sharing household tasks and working on the flower beds. Sarah developed into quite the gardener. She's probably surpassed me now, especially with growing vegetables.

I was her coach for Colton's birth. How things have changed since I gave birth. Birthing rooms are now the norm and large enough to accommodate everything to assess a newborn right in the room, with plenty of room for the coach. Midwives are more common. There's no question about rooming in. Lactation specialists are there to assist with breastfeeding.

Colton was in the NICU for a short period. I would drop Sarah at the hospital before heading to work and pick her up when she was ready to go home. Today's neonatal layettes would have accommodated even Jimmy at nine pounds. Strange to have a newborn in the house. I pitched in, but mostly I was a grandmother. I finished his quilt when he was about six months old.

A couple of years later, Kenny and April had a daughter, Kinley. I drove to Charlotte to see her at a day old. A few weeks later, I went back down to lend a hand. There's always so much to do with a newborn. I try to carry on the family tradition of women helping each other during times like these. I know I always appreciated Momma's help. Besides, I like all the cuddles.

Before Jon came home, Sarah, Colton, and I flew to Galveston for Catherine's wedding. The flights were horrendous; Colton cried most of the time we were in the air. He was probably picking up my discomfort with flying. Sarah rented a condo and a car for us. Colton I and went to the beach even though it was a little cool while Sarah attended to her duties as Matron of Honor. The wedding venue and décor were beautiful. Colton was precious in his little seer sucker suit. Catherine and Corey were stunning in their wedding finery.

Sarah and Jon moved to Fayetteville. They eventually bought a house in White Oak. We all pitched in to help empty the apartment in Fayetteville. Keith and I stayed a few days to help them get settled.

During this time, Jimmy, Kenny, Sarah, and I began long talks "about how to solve the world's problems". Kenny and I have become notorious in the family for talking into the wee hours. Obviously, we can't solve the world's problems. Still, for each of us, these talks have helped sharpen our awareness of events taking place in the world and introduce us different ways of thinking.

I was also fortunate to be working with several young Black women. Our discussions helped me grow a great deal and sharpen my perceptions of the world. We talked honestly with each other. More of us need to talk honestly.

I always wanted to help everyone who needed help and felt bad because I couldn't, even as I knew it was impossible. These talks with my children and my coworkers at ACT, over the years, helped me reconcile my idealist self and realistic self. So that I could accept helping just one person. Hopefully, the ripples would spread to others.

33

COVID-19

In March 2020, I was already feeling the strain of being the only nurse on our ACT team while trying to help the social workers with case management. A corporate decision downsized to us to a small team the previous October, but we were still providing care to the same number of people. I struggled to complete annual health screenings that helped our clients stay abreast of their medical conditions.

The novel coronavirus, eventually named COVID-19, certainly wreaked havoc with everything throughout the country. It's impact on our ACT team was devastating. It fractured our delivery of care as we went to telehealth visits when possible. Isolation gear placed a barrier between us and our individual clients. Our morning meetings took place on Zoom. I stopped holding wellness classes to reduce the risk of spreading the virus. I stopped doing annual screening because of the closeness required.

Regarding the virus, no one was sure about anything. For years, I had in-serviced my team members about various health conditions so they could better understand how our clients' medical conditions might affect their ability to function. Now, as they looked to me for answers, I had none to give. Just the bulletins put out by the health department and what we heard on the news. These sources did not really add much to our knowledge base. People were sick. People were dying. According to the news, there were not enough ventilators or isolation gear for healthcare providers.

Is the virus transmitted by droplet? Is it airborne? My training told me it was airborne. The Center for Disease Control (CDC) waffled with their recommendations. No one knew for sure. Either way, we needed more masks, and my usual supplier only had a limited quantity. I ordered what I could. After my initial order, my supplier limited the amount I could order as they struggled to supply everyone and then, even they could not get masks.

On a weekend, I made three cotton masks for each member of my team. I wanted to make more but couldn't find elastic in nearby stores and had to order it from Amazon. It took two weeks for the elastic to be delivered.

I encouraged my coworkers to wear their cotton masks but to be sure to wash them after each day's wear. Already, there was war raging in my head about infection control. Ideally, we should have disposable masks that are thrown away after each encounter. Now we are wearing the same mask all day. If we were careful not to touch the outside of the mask, we would be okay. Wouldn't we? I could only hope. I in-serviced my coworkers about donning and removing masks. Once my Amazon order arrived, I made enough masks for our ACT team in Greensboro, our administrative staff and family members that didn't sew.

Governor Cooper established several emergency measures in North Carolina. This included asking people to stay home except for essential things, stay six feet apart and wear a face mask in public. Hospitals stopped all elective procedures and visitation. Businesses implemented various COVID precautions to operate. Some precautions included decreasing the number of patrons based on the building's square footage and having a method for sanitizing shopping carts and other things in the store. People lined up outside grocery stores. Stores marked entrances and check-out lines to encourage people to remain six feet apart. Some restaurants stayed in business by serving takeout. The state government considered bars, gyms, event centers and movie theaters nonessential. Travel bans disrupted businesses and family gatherings. At work, the corporate office issued letters declaring our status as essential workers for us to carry. As things worked out, I never had to show the letter to travel for work.

All these measures sparked debates not only across the nation, but within my family. Some family members felt the measures were going too far. I led with my "public health gut" and felt most measures were necessary to keep North Carolina from experiencing the huge number of deaths as seen in New York and other states. The impact on businesses was tremendous with many going under. However, our local healthcare system was strained but never overwhelmed.

Several times a day, I visited the websites for the CDC and the North Carolina Department of Health and Human Services (NCDHHS) as I tried to find answers for all my questions. All the bulletins urged us to wear a mask, stay six feet apart and wash your hands frequently. Being a nurse meant I was often much closer to my clients than six feet. *How do I keep from spreading the virus wearing the same isolation gear to see multiple clients?* NCDHHS listed the COVID case count by county. COVID was spreading towards Alamance County from the eastern, more densely populated counties.

Personally, I my depression worsened. After talking with the psychiatrist at work, I started taking Trintellix. It worked well without undo side effects. It caused some nausea, but eating small snacks during the day counteracted this side effect.

Eventually, we got N95 masks, procedure masks, face shields and isolation gowns. Because of limited supplies, my coworkers used procedure masks and face shields. Our team handed out masks to our clients. We reserved the N95 masks and isolation gowns for me as I had to work within our clients' personal space. Initially, I had five N95 masks. One for each day of the work week. At the end of each day, I would put the mask in a paper bag, put it on top of a cabinet and let it rest. I prayed any viruses would die before I wore the mask again in five days. The

CDC felt nurses in hospitals could let their mask rest for three days before reusing it.

Isolation gear involves a plastic or impermeable fabric-like gown, a face mask covering your nose and mouth and goggles, or a face shield. You look like an alien. Even worse, the face shield resembles riot gear. Although I called my clients to give them an advanced notice about the isolation gear I was wearing, the gear disturbed some of my clients.

"Is that you, Nurse Sherry?" a client asks as they open the door.

"Yes, it's me. Sorry about the get up, but I'm trying to be sure that I don't bring the virus into your home."

"Thanks for that. But we can't have you getting sick either. I need you to come see me. I'm glad you have the right stuff to wear. Better that we all be safe."

One client was so disturbed by the face shield, I stopped wearing it for his visits.

"You don't look right wearing that. You look like an alien from outer space. I can't get it out of my mind."

"Okay." I remove the face shield. "How's this? Can you tell it's me now? Can I come in?"

"Yeah, I've seen my doctors like that. Come on in and give my shot, Nurse Sherry."

Since several of my clients dealt with persist delusions and hallucinations, I'm surprised that more of them did not have difficulty with the isolation gear. Eventually, my husband found goggles at Lowe's that would fit over my glasses, and I stopped wearing the face shield at all. Overall, most clients saw the isolation gear for what it was—an attempt to keep everyone safe.

I had a routine for disinfecting everything. Before I left a client's home, I wiped down my scales, stethoscope, thermometer, and any other reusable diagnostic equipment. Then I would spray down the bags, my goggles and isolation gown before reentering the van after a client visit. I would repeat the disinfecting process when I returned to the office, spraying down my company van and everything in it.

In the world of infection control, if a dirty item touches a clean one, they are now both dirty. I sometimes forgot what was clean and what was dirty. Infection control does not have a five-second rule. Sometimes I would stop and restart several times before I was sure I had disinfected every surface. At the office we joked the virus didn't have a chance: disinfectant spray would bring about our demise.

Although I still visited reliable websites, I stopped watching the news. Pictures of body bags in refrigerated trailers and nurses improvising isolation gear haunted me. I couldn't get them out of my mind. If this is happening in our big cities, what will happen here in a smaller town with fewer resources?

If the questions surrounding my work weren't disturbing enough, both my daughter and daughter-in-law were pregnant. How would this killer virus affect them and their unborn child? No one could say.

My family was now only texting and talking on the phone. I missed them. We usually got together once a month. I stopped shopping. I could no longer go to the fitness center. It was closed, as it wasn't "essential" under North Carolina's emergency mandate. My husband began doing all the shopping since I was out in the community five days a week.

Then there were the shortages, hand sanitizer, disinfectants, toilet paper and other paper products. Some people panicked and simply bought up everything they could find. Other shortages occurred because of problems in the supply chain as workers became sick. Stores limited the number of cleaning and paper products you could purchase at a time. Eventually, there were limits on how much meat you could buy at a time. At work, my regional director took over ordering supplies. Mystic, a local distillery, began making hand sanitizer, and our director purchased some. Just as I was about to run out of toilet paper at home, BJ's had "healthcare provider's hours". They had toilet paper on the day I shopped.

Globally, people were calling nurses heroes. It has always made me uncomfortable when people do this. Nurses chose their profession for several reasons and they're all personal. Nursing *is* a demanding profession. But calling us heroes? I understand most people are trying to express gratitude for something they can't do and couldn't do. But to me, calling us heroes makes us one dimensional. I have professional knowledge. Calling me a hero ignores the professional skills that allow me to provide lifesaving treatments. It also ignores my humanity. It makes it easier for facilities and institutions to ignore the fact that most nurses are overworked and underpaid.

The deaths of Breonna Taylor and George Floyd at the hands of police officers brought our country's racial disparities to the forefront. Alamance County saw protests over a confederate statue at a historic courthouse. So many senseless deaths. So much pain. Why can't we just see people as human beings? Why do we repeat the same mistakes? Unrest swept the country.

By the end of May, my family got together for a cookout. It was wonderful to see and hug everyone. Shortly afterwards, my youngest son again brought up his proposal to purchase a house for Keith and me. We went back and forth for a bit, but he finally convinced us this was part of his financial plan, as the house would be an investment for him. He would buy the house and we would make the mortgage payments.

Near the end of June, Kenny, Keith, and I went to look at a few houses. It was odd with the COVID restrictions. Few people on the road. No one wanted to touch anything. Of course, we wore our masks. There weren't that many houses in our price range available. We looked at a few but they weren't quite it. After a quick phone call, our agent took us to see a house that wasn't on the market yet but would be soon.

Walking in through the front door, I knew this was the house for us. They had renovated the interior within the last three years. Except for the living room, there were hardwood floors throughout. Right away I could see us living in this house, the grandkids running through the house and the big, fenced backyard. No more worry about Coco being out in the road. There was no question where the Christmas tree would go. Kenny and April put in an offer and after a brief dance of offer and counteroffer, the house was ours. I felt like someone on a TV show--- getting my dream house.

A flurry of packing began. Sarah came up from White Oak and did an amazing job. Because we pack the same way, I could say "pack this room" and head off to work. When I came home, she had boxes packed and labeled so I knew what was in them. I could jump into packing without missing a beat.

In the middle of this, I received a call to let me know my youngest brother, Martin, had died. He had finally succumbed to heart disease. We had grown apart over the last few years. Martin developed views which were polar opposites of mine, and we never found a way to "agree to disagree". With COVID, there was no way to attend the funeral.

This time, Keith and I hired a moving company to transport the boxes once we had everything packed. Everyone's work schedules, along with Sarah's and April's pregnancies, made this a simpler way to go. Before the movers delivered our household goods, Kenny and Jimmy came over and helped set up a gazebo on the patio of the new house. Keith added an outdoor fan to its ceiling. We sure needed it moving the in the middle of July. I prohibited Sarah and April from further help with the move. I felt moving was one thing that they didn't need. My sister and her husband came down from Virginia to help me get settled.

With Terry's help, the kitchen was functional on the first day. We dug and potted up my roses, cone plants, Asiatic lilies and irises. This would keep them alive until I could replant them at the new house. Keith and Doug set up the grill, hung curtain rods, and got the laundry room functional.

Within the first week, Keith had a load of dirt delivered to the backyard. Without trees, we didn't really have a place for our bird feeders. Bird watching was such a big part of our relaxation, he created an area for a crepe myrtle, a Little Gem Magnolia and the flowers. Kenny jokingly called it Tweet-Tweet Island. The name stuck.

Of course, Keith and I continued working throughout the move. His business had been doing well for the last several years. For me, the on-call rotation got shorter with fewer people in the office. The calls to our crisis line got more intense. Some of our newer clients were more ill and other's illness became exacerbated by everything happening in the world. At work, we encouraged people to decrease their time spent watching the news.

I had been having some trouble with urinary incontinence. Although few people talk about it, urinary incontinence is common in women who had large babies or who did a lot of lifting in their jobs. Either of those things can lead to a prolapse, which presses on the bladder. I was spending way too much time figuring out how far away I was from a bathroom. I felt I was too many years post-menopausal to be wearing a pad again. Several weeks of physical therapy were helpful. My physical therapist and I hoped I could avoid surgery.

This was an odd time of highs and lows. COVID and unrest going through the country were absolute lows. I was in my home, my "I'm never moving again home", and my family was well. Those were absolute highs. Even though I was again having trouble sleeping, I was immensely grateful for all I had.

34

COVID Hits Home

Leaving a client's home, suddenly I didn't feel well. Beads of sweat rolled down my face and neck, creating uncomfortable pools wherever my clothing gathered against my skin. *It's 85 degrees and I'm in full isolation gear. No wonder I'm sweating. Just get in the van and turn on the AC.*

During the twenty-minute ride back to the office, I'm not feeling better, and the sweat continues to drip down my face. *That damned AC is out again. Have to get the van in the shop.* By the time I arrive at the office, I know I'm sick and can't blame the sweat on faulty air conditioning. I would have bet my paycheck on the diagnosis.

Thankfully, no one was in the office when I returned. I disinfected the van and my gear as usual. Once in the med room, I checked my temperature. The thermometer blinked red with a 102 reading. As I made a few preparations to be out of the office for a while, I called my supervisor and gave her the bad news.

"Hey, I'm going to get tested in just a few minutes. I've got a temp of 102. Pretty sure this will be a positive test."

"Oh, no Miss Sherry. Go take care of yourself."

"I've got meds pulled and ready for a week. I'll disinfect my way out the door."

"Just go. Let me know when you hear something. I'll be praying for you. Let us know if you need anything."

"Okay, I will. Thanks."

I called Keith while I was waiting in line to get tested and gave him the news. Once I was home, we set up the spare room as a sickroom. By the time we were through converting the couch to a bed and getting it made up, I had depleted my energy reserves and crawled into bed. I remember admonishing Keith to change the sheets on our bed and disinfect the kitchen as I fell asleep.

A few days later, I got the news that my test was positive. A doctor from the hospital called to give me instructions for home care and to remind me that COVID-19 was reportable to the Health Department. I called work and made my supervisor aware of the positive test results. As this was Friday, I didn't expect to hear from the public health nurse until Monday.

The nurse called on Saturday. After going over my contact list, she gave me instructions for home care; take Tylenol for fever, drink plenty of fluids and use a separate bathroom from the rest of the household, if possible. She also told me that should I have trouble breathing or have the feeling of impending doom, I should go to the hospital right away. *I knew COVID was serious, but I hadn't heard the words "impending doom" since nursing school. My brain ran to pulmonary emboli, strokes and other forms of sudden death.*

We talked on the phone every day for a week. The health department sent out a COVID care kit complete with thermometer, masks, hand sanitizer and disinfecting wipes as well as written care instructions. Contactless delivery, of course.

"Good morning, Sherry. How are you today?" My nurse asked when she called on Monday.

"I'm hanging in here. My temperature keeps spiking. Let me get my notebook and I'll give you the rundown."

"You're such a nurse! Writing things down."

"I'm so tired and I sleep in spurts. I'm afraid I'll forget something."

"That's as expected."

She called every day. On Friday, she changed things up. "For the next while, text me your vitals before noon. If something changes, call me. If you don't text, I'll call."

Keith cooked and brought meals to my room for me. I didn't want him coming into the room. So, we talked with him standing in the doorway and me on the far side of the room. We already used separate bathrooms. Nothing tasted or smelled good, not even coffee. I made myself eat—fried egg sandwiches on toast or chicken noodle soup was about all I could handle. I had lower GI symptoms, nausea, and diarrhea, rather than respiratory symptoms. The Trintellix exacerbated the nausea, so I stopped taking it. Keith kept my water glass full and made sure that I sat in my chair for a while.

Just a few days after my diagnosis, Kenny and April welcomed Adalynn into the world. I didn't see her until she was three weeks old. Sarah set up her nursery without me. I so badly wanted to be there for both families, but could only wait out the course of the illness and remain in isolation.

The stories about COVID nightmares are real. Realizing high fevers cause delirium, which can cause nightmares, did not make things any better. The worst of my nightmares took place in a hospital room. The lights are bright white. I squint against the brightness; try to understand what is happening. My family is circled around my bed. I know they are all here. I can't see their faces clearly. Just their tears reflecting the light. I hear a doctor talking, "We should intubate her." I panic. *Don't let them do this to me!* I'm yelling, but no one can hear me. They're all holding onto each other. Their crying gets louder. Keith tells the doctor, "No, she wouldn't want that". I'm yelling, trying to tell them I'm okay, but no one can hear me. I wake up and realize I'm home.

After the dreams, many times, I was afraid to go to sleep. Afraid I wouldn't wake up. Afraid I would dream again. I usually try to face my fears, figure out the trigger and reason out a way to deal with it. But I couldn't this time. Actually, I knew the trigger. COVID has killed people. It didn't matter that I knew what caused the nightmares.

Finally, I confessed my fear to Keith. His simple "You're strong. You're going to be okay." made everything alright. I slept. I kept waking up.

All we could do was treat my symptoms and prevent secondary infection. I had read nurses were encouraging hospital patients to sleep on their stomachs to improve their respiratory function; I slept on my stomach. Every few hours I made myself get up for at least a half hour. I did deep breathing exercises to keep my airways clear. Reading took up some of my time. I re-watched Call the Midwife starting from the first season. I spent a lot of time watching the birds on Tweet-Tweet Island, thinking, feeling grateful. Keith planted my roses and other plants we brought from our old house, knowing I wouldn't get to them for a while. The white and yellow Knock-Out roses were precious to me, but nothing like the peace rose. The peace rose is a long stem rose. It's bud forms in a pale yellow. As it unfolds, there are blushes of pink at each petal's edge. Family, friends, and coworkers called to make sure I knew they loved me.

I scribbled thoughts into notebooks. The American Nurses Association had proclaimed 2020 the "Year of the Nurse" and put out a call for nurses to share their stories. I often shook my head at the irony of a global pandemic occurring during this time. I wanted to submit something to them, but trying to script a three-minute video was not something I was comfortable doing. Besides, I'd rather write an article than film a video.

Things that had hovered around my consciousness for the last few years became clearer. Having time without distractions gave me time to think about where my life was going and how I wanted to spend my time. What I genuinely wanted to do was to visit my family without regard for a work schedule or how short staffed the office would be while I was out; to sew and quilt; to write. After talking with Keith, I decided I would retire at the end of the year instead of waiting until June.

Still in quarantine and bored one day, I remembered seeing different writers' workshops sponsored by the public library and being upset that their timing never fit in with mine. Feeling that I needed to do something besides scribble in my notebooks before life overtook me again, I searched the internet. I didn't find any offerings. I was hoping for at least a Zoom workshop.

By chance, I found the website for the Burlington Writer's Club (BWC). BWC has been around for a long time. I was hesitant, but contacted the president about the October meeting. Her response was prompt and enthusiastic. I added the date to my planner.

I was unbelievably tired. It wasn't so much shortness of breath as a lack of energy. Even as I felt better, something as simple as doing a load of laundry exhausted me. After showering and washing my hair, I had to rest for about an hour before I could blow dry my hair. My public health nurse extended my quarantine because I was so exhausted.

At the end of my quarantine, I wondered how I would function at work. With a note from my doctor, I took another week off from work. By the time I returned, I had been out for a month, and I still didn't have my former stamina.

Although I had a mild case of COVID and my recovery was relatively quick, having COVID brought my personal mortality front and center. I'm thankful fatigue was my only lasting complication and I'm fortunate I can work to bring some of my reflections into being.

35

Back to Work

I spent my first day back in the office to figure out where we were with injections, get updates on clients' statuses and try to catch up. Nurses from our Greensboro office administered injections while I was out. I was grateful they did a good job with documentation. It made the process much easier.

Emotionally, I wasn't ready to be at work. We still had Zoom meetings instead of our usual face-to-face morning meeting. While everyone was happy for me to be back, I had trouble reconnecting. Probably because mentally, I had already said goodbye. Most people were making telehealth calls from home. It wasn't so bad when I was in the office alone, but when someone else was in the office, my anxiety kicked into high gear.

The workdays were hectic as I juggled seeing patients and scheduling COVID vaccinations for our clients. Fortunately, I had begun patient teaching about the vaccine as it was being developed. Now, it was just a matter of seeing who wanted the vaccine and scheduling the appointment. The ACT team would provide transportation. All our clients who wanted a vaccine got one.

I just kept trying to get through the days. BWC put out a call for submissions to the 65th Anniversary Anthology. The piece I was writing, "A Bend in the Road", dealt with my experiences during the COVID and would be my submission to the anthology. It limped along. I was so tired

I didn't do much after work. My doctor felt my fatigue was a symptom of long COVID and eventually my energy levels would improve.

The weekend was for housework. I struggled to give myself permission to take a nap. I know all the rejuvenating effects of sleep, but I have always felt it was a waste of time. I longed to once more be that person who only needed four or five hours of sleep a night. For years, I was that person, but no more.

Because of COVID, Sarah had not really met her neighbors, so other than me or Jon's mom, there was no one to watch Colton for even a few hours. Jon's mom couldn't switch her schedule easily, as she was the primary caregiver for Jon's grandmother. The original plan was for me to meet Sarah, Jon, and Colton at the hospital when she was in labor. I would then take Colton back to their house. I was so tired most of the time I doubted my ability to get there quickly and still have energy for Colton.

Halloween passed without Sarah going into active labor. Talking with her on the phone, we amended the plan. It sounded like Lilith might join us on Monday or Tuesday. I called my supervisor to activate my time off. Sunday morning, I drove down to White Oak. Hopefully, I'd get used to Colton's routine and get a night's rest before being responsible for Colton.

Lilith entered our world without problems. Because of COVID, if Jon left the hospital, he would have to stay out until noon the next day. Also, Colton and I couldn't visit. He got to video call Sarah and see his little sister. It was a great time for the two of us. We fed the chickens and played baseball in the side yard.

Just a few weeks later, we were all together for a family Thanksgiving. For the first time in many years, I cooked a Thanksgiving meal for just the immediate family---not the usual 17 to 21. Best Thanksgiving we had in years. The cooking was easier. But the best part was that we had more time to engage with each other. To be there in the moment.

Returning to work after Thanksgiving, I told my supervisor of my plan to retire at the end of December and that I would give her my official letter of resignation December first. I agreed to work part-time with no on call until they found a new nurse. I could feel the weight lifting from my shoulders.

When the vaccines were first offered, I was ambivalent about getting one. Its development was moving too quickly from what I could see. Fortunately, through work, I attended a few online seminars regarding the development of the vaccines, which helped dispel some of my concerns. They also explained North Carolina's plan to roll out vaccine delivery based on an individual's risk of developing serious complications should they contract COVID-19.

In December, I took the first dose of my vaccine. The first in my family to receive it, I joked with them "So far so good, I haven't grown a new arm or become magnetic. It must be okay". It wasn't an attempt to demean those with serious concerns about the vaccine's safety, just my nurse's dark humor as I tried to provide reassurance to everyone.

Also in December, I received word the BWC accepted my piece, "A Bend in the Road", for its anthology. Publication would occur in 2021. Being a published author put me on cloud nine. My family and BWC inspired me to keep writing. I entered a piece in the BWC spring writer's contest.

The first weekend of April found Sarah, Keith, and me at Greensboro Shrub nursery, along with Colton and Lily. As often happens in North Carolina, we entered a cold spell right before Sarah and the children arrived. Bundled in winter coats and wearing gloves, we walked through the greenhouses and along rows of plants lining the dirt roads through the nursery to make our selections.

My goal was to replace many of the plants that I had left at my previous house. Sarah was buying a few blueberry bushes and hostas as well. We easily found a bleeding heart for the nod to my grandma. The hostas were harder to choose. So many varieties. Finally, I decided on a patriot, a variegated variety with large portions of pale yellow, and a stiletto, it's medium green leaves have a narrow knife blade like shape. But the name always makes me think of the tall stiletto heels that Momma, Sarah, and

I loved. I also bought several varieties of cone flowers and astilbe. Still suffering from post-COVID fatigue, sometimes I stood near the end of a group of plants watching Colton as he ran splashing through the mud puddles while Sarah continued her search. Seeing Colton turn a little blue as he became soaked from his water play brought an end to the plant hunt. Although his teeth were chattering, only the promise of hot chocolate convinced Colton to get into the car quickly. He was having too much fun splashing in the puddles.

Although the weather was still cold, the next day we were out in the flower beds right after breakfast. When you've been doing it for years, getting plants in the ground is not that complicated. However, my flower beds were nothing but packed red clay and there was no time for amending the entire bed. Sarah loaded my green canvas wagon with bags of garden soil and pulled it up next to the beds. I hadn't had my surgery yet, so lifting was out of the question for me. Our plan was to dig a hole much larger than each plant needed, fill it with gardening soil, set in the plant and finally, fill in with more garden soil.

After we arranged the plants throughout the garden, we started planting. As long as I could sit on my gardening camp stool, I could plant the smaller one quart pots. Sarah put in all the plants in gallon containers since they required digging with a shovel. We worked most of the day, in between taking care of the children. Lily was only about six months old. By the time we finished, my flower garden had a good beginning for the eclectic English cottage garden I love.

Sarah had the hardest job. Like Momma, when I helped her, I spent more time looking after Colton running through the yard, listening for Lily on the monitor and saying "yes, that looks good" when Sarah asked if a placement was okay, than actually putting plants in the ground. My life had come full circle. In some ways, it's wonderful. It's harder in other ways, like accepting the fact that doing some things is more difficult than it was ten years ago. Intellectually, I recognize how aging affects your body. I'm still working on the acceptance part. I also realize I'll probably be working on this for the rest of my life.

The piece I entered for the BWC Writer's contest received an honorable mention. Elation could not come close to describing my mood. I was floating on a cloud. Someone else, other writers, thought my work was good. I wanted to write all the time. Pre-Covid, there would have been a banquet at which members could read their work. Because of COVID concerns, we had a Zoom meeting. Although I was nervous about reading my work to anyone, much less fellow authors, I read my piece "Seeds". It was the story of the winding road I took to becoming a nurse.

I never resumed taking my antidepressant. As I continued to recover, I found my mood remained positive. Yes, there were down moods, but nothing my coping skills couldn't handle.

When I wasn't working, I was writing or reading about writing. Initially, I thought I'd write the stories my children wanted me to tell and submit them to different magazines or contests. Maybe later, I would gather them into a collection, I thought. In short order, I decided to just write this book. I set myself a daily word count goal and stayed at my laptop until I met it. Some days I struggled, but other days I soared.

It took until May for my replacement to be hired. I stayed onboard long enough to train her. The office gave me a wonderful party. While I knew I would miss my coworkers and clients, I looked forward to spending my time doing what I wanted and doing it at my own pace.

36

Epilogue

I had surgery at the end of July 2021. Nothing life threatening, pelvic floor reconstruction surgery to take care of the prolapse. I was anxious about the anesthesia. I still don't like the idea of not being in control of myself. I had the surgery on a Thursday and came home with a Foley catheter. Fortunately, I knew this was a possibility and purchased a few loose dresses beforehand. Sarah and her children came and stayed through the weekend. I had confessed my biggest concern was keeping my pain medications straight since they make me loopier than a roller coaster. My sweet daughter woke up every six hours to bring me pain medication for the first two nights. Her being here also made Keith feel comfortable about going to work. The surgery made such a difference in my quality of life.

During my recovery period, days flowed by, one blending into the other. Sitting in the sun watching the birds at the feeders. Going to doctor's appointments. This was not what I had envisioned for retirement. I began using my planner again. Just to help me give some structure to my days. I still wasn't used to not having to get up for work. Or just taking things at my pace. Life while I was working meant always pushing through with projects before going back to work on Monday or risk losing the impetus to finish them. The problem now became prioritizing everything I wanted to do.

At the end of September, I received a call from my old employer. The nurse had quit abruptly, and they needed someone to help with injections. There was no hesitation in meeting my new salary and scheduling requirements. When I reported in, I found corporate was closing the Burlington office. I wound up working four weeks to help transfer our clients to other providers. The administrative assistant and I were the only ones remaining in the office. Transferring clients to other services reminded me so much of closing the facility in Chapel Hill. Corporate issued deadlines without realizing how long the process took. Even when an agency accepted a client, it could take a couple of weeks to complete the transition. While I appreciated the welcome I received from my clients, this experience confirmed that I had made the right decision to retire from nursing and pursue other interests.

Over the years, I learned ways to deal with my depression and past trauma. Others find they need the help of a counselor or therapist. I've learned what keeps me mentally healthy. It is important to break the cycle of abuse, be it physical, emotional, or sexual. My mother grew up in a home where the man ruled the house and punished severely, often physically. Despite all her wonderful traits, Momma could not pick a husband. They were all abusive. Her own punishments were harsh. Early in life, I realized violence begets violence. Understanding what emotional abuse was and overcoming it took longer.

I don't have all the answers, but I believe we need to listen not only to our hearts and minds, but to our bodies as well. We are healthier when these three things stay connected. It is an ongoing journey. I still don't understand why some of us are more resilient than others. Something tells me I'll be trying to answer that question for the rest of my days.

The younger me thought I should have accomplished so many things by a particular age. The quilt of my life, as I imagined it, would encompass triangle shapes forming squares, following straight lines. But it didn't turn out that way. My life has been more like a crazy quilt. It's made up of different shapes adapted, as life me brought fresh challenges. My experiences are the embroidery which highlight sections of my quilt. The ups, the downs, twists, and turns all resulted in a quilt uniquely my own.

I would not have written this book if it had not been for the persistent requests from my children, in particular Kenny and Sarah. They listened patiently as I worked through different sections. Often they added their own memories of events, adding layers to the story.

Keith provided invaluable encouragement, from his "I'm glad you're writing" as I sat in front of my laptop to "Your story is important". He helped me stay focused and helped me believe in myself.

Finally, the Burlington Writers Club helped me see how to get the words scribbled in a notebook out into the world. The ACC Critique group provided invaluable feedback as I presented portions of this book for review in our meetings.

www.ingramcontent.com/pod-product-compliance
Lightning Source LLC
Chambersburg PA
CBHW060515130626
46553CB00002B/510

* 9 7 9 8 2 1 8 0 3 0 7 6 6 *